OPTICIANRY: THE PRACTICE AND THE ART
Volume II The Science of Opticianry

A Programmed Text
Second Edition
by

William A. Borover
Master Optician

Illustrated by Wendi Borover

GRACIE ENTERPRISES, INC.—PUBLISHER

First Printing — August, 1982
Second Printing — July, 1987

Library of Congress Number 81-82152
ISBN 09606398-2-9
O.U.R. Number 1033

Other Books by William A. Borover:
Opticianry, The Practice and the Art, Volume I — Introduction to Dispensing
Opticianry, The Practice and the Art, Volume III — The Dynamics of Dispensing
Opticianry, The Practice and the Art, Volume IV — The Business of Opticianry
The Irate Patient — Audio Cassette Seminar

Published by: Gracie Enterprises, Inc.
P.O Box 506
Chula Vista, California
92012-0506
(619) 421-8055

TO YOU, THE READER

Now that you have read *Volume I* of this series, I welcome you back. As you will see, the programmed instructional format you so enjoyed in *Volume I* continues in this Book: *OPTICIANRY — THE PRACTICE AND THE ART: VOL. II, The Science of Opticianry*.

THE SCIENCE OF OPTICIANRY is designed to provide you with the next level: a working knowledge of the Rx as it relates both to the frame and the patient. The exercises have been especially prepared in increasing degrees of difficulty, thus allowing you to apply a previous chapter's knowledge to a new concept. The number of self-tests have also been increased to allow you more practice with a particular subject.

You will also notice the improved programming format which will facilitate reading.

Please let me know how you enjoyed *Volume II*. You know, I believe these may be the best frames you'll never wear.

— Bill Borover

This Book is for you . . .

THE DOCTOR:	As a training manual for your assistants, as a resource, for your library, as an overview of Opticianry as it may pertain to your practice.
THE ASSISTANT, AIDE:	As a learning device for office personnel, as a bridge to better understanding of the dispenser's role; lensometry, the prescription, the patient.
THE SCHOOL:	As a classroom text, as a workbook, as a library resource.
THE LAB:	As an overview of the Optician's role, the Rx order, the finishing laboratory's procedures.
THE REP:	As an introduction to the science of Opticianry, criteria for frame selection, the product, the prescription.
THE OPTICIAN:	As an effective training manual for the dispenser, a concise guide to the prescription, the frame, and the patient.

Acknowledgements

Thank you, Mom and Dad, from one William.

Thank you, Mom and Dad, for one Wendi.

Thank you, Brenda, once again, for your help in putting my scribbling into words.

Thank you, Mike DiSanto, F.N.A.O., for your kind collaboration.

A special thank-you to Irwin Vogel, Professor of Ophthalmic Dispensing, Cañada College.

TO MY WIFE, WENDI,

without whose love, understanding,
and enthusiasm this book also
would not have been possible.

About The Author

William A. Borover, F.N.A.O., Master Optician, speaker, lecturer, author, was born in Cleveland, Ohio, in 1939. Before entering the ophthalmic field, he spent a number of years as a professional magician. Bill began apprenticing in an optical wholesale lab in 1959 and thereafter entered into retail dispensing. His experience in Opticianry provided ophthalmic environments at the clinical, industrial and retail levels.

Returning to the University, Bill earned a B.A. in education and became an education area specialist for the Cuyahoga Community College Ophthalmic (Opticianry) Dispensing Technology Program. He helped implement and coordinate Ohio's first Opticianry school program and became Program Leader and Head Instructor. Moving to Southern California in 1978, Bill became Executive Director of Eye Physicians Medical Surgical Center, Chula Vista, CA. In July of 1986, Bill began to devote full time to Gracie Enterprises as Executive Director of the Ophthalmic Practice Improvement division where he currently works. He lives in San Diego with his wife, Wendi, and their two collies.

Among his other credits are: Past Trustee, The Ohio Society of Dispensing Opticians; Fellow, The International Academy of Opticianry; Fellow, The National Academy of Opticianry; Master of Ophthalmic Optics, The American Board of Opticianry; Charter and Certified Optician, The American Board of Opticianry; Past Commissioner, The Commission of Opticianry Accreditation; Faculty, The San Diego City College; Life Teaching Credential, The California Community Colleges; Registered Contact Lens Dispenser; The National Committee of Contact Lens Examiners; Member, The Contact Lens Society of America; Spectacle-Contact Lens Dispensing Optician; The State of Ohio Optical Dispensers Board; Member, Medical Research Associates Advisory Panel; Past Education Chairman, The California Society of Dispensing Opticians; Member, The Opticians Association of America; Member, The Editorial Review Board; The National Academy of Opticianry; Faculty; Optifair, Board of Directors; The Society For Office Based Surgery, Published articles: The Optical Index, 20/20, The Dispensing Optician, Optical Management. Bill Borover has been a popular contributor to local, state and national educational ophthalmic programs.

Preface to the First Edition

I can vividly remember back to the early days when the why's were unexplained. The techniques of dispensing were empirically established; things were done because that's the way they were always done. Books on ophthalmic dispensing were as scarce as locksets the more esoteric treatises were foreboding. For the earnest Optician who sought the answers to the why's and wherefore's, the revelations came slowly, sometimes painfully as running too many right eyes. Secrets were passed down by word of mouth; jealously guarded like some clandestine conspiracy, thus obviating the most important participant of eye care: The Patient.

There were plenty of texts on geometric and physical optics, but few addressed themselves to an organized step-by-step procedure for the dispensing Optician. It was then, as I read through the available literature, that I realized there was a need to teach THE BEGINNING. Where does one start? I decided I would create, with a series of volumes, the "bridge" to the more advanced literature.

And so, it is with this purpose: to clarify, to simplify, to share, that I have labored, hoping above all, that the perpetuation of OPTICIANRY: ITS PRACTICE AND ITS ART may be assured through learning and application, through enthusiasm and love for the patient.

TO YOU, THE READER —

HOW TO USE THIS BOOK:

A. The reader reads a small amount of information (usually equal to a paragraph).

B. The author asks a question about what you just read (Yes, this book actually talks to you).

C. The reader WRITES the answer in the space provided and then . . . turns the page to check the answer with the author's correct answer. Then, the pattern repeats: more info, another question or reference to an illustration, write the answer, turn the page and check the answer.

To accommodate this writing and page-turning, this book's format is a little different from most texts; it's written in sections or "frames" that look like this:

Answer 32. (Author's correct answer in this space)

. . . .

Frame 33. (Information here)

(Questions here) (Illustrations here)

____

(Reader writes answer in this space)

There are two sections, or frames, to a page. To make this programmed text even easier, the reader starts on Page 1, at the top, reads, writes, and turns the page. The next section, or frame, is found at the top right-hand side of THAT page and so on. After the reader has read thru all the top right-hand frames, the instructions are to return to Page 1 and read and write in the bottom right-hand frames. This programmed method continues and builds on information easily learned on all right-hand pages, until the reader reaches the last bottom right-hand frame; then the same process continues on the left-hand pages. Try it! It works!

Enjoy learning from the easiest textbook you ever read . . . . Gracie Enterprises, Inc.
Publisher

Table of Contents

Answer 756. The Beginning

Frame 757.

CHAPTER 1
INSTRUCTIONS

PLEASE TURN TO **FRAME 758,** ON THE TOP OF PAGE 3

Answer 894. Go to Frame 895.

Frame 895. Your chart should look like this. Check your answers and turn to the bottom of Page 3, Frame 896.

'B' box	Wanted O.C. Height	Decentration	Direction
A) 46	25	2.0 mm.	Up
B) 52	23	3.0 mm.	Down
C) 57	26	2.5 mm.	Down
D) 62	31	0.0	0

Answer 1032. Freebie — Any answer is correct!

Frame 1033. This is a special frame. Lets face it, this business of optics for education is demanding, but it is the only way we Opticians can be judged as professionally competent. So, take a break, get a grip, sip a beverage, hug a loved one, and let us toast... Good Reading And Continuing Instructional Education.

TO GRACIE!

THEN. . .CONTINUE ON TO
THE TOP OF PAGE 4, **FRAME 1034**

Answer 1170. Up (You seem to have it!)

Frame 1171. The lens for Frame 1170 then, needs to be decentered 4 mm. in **and** 2 mm. up. Study the representation of 4 in and 2 up on the graph in this frame.

As you can see it is important to notate the front or back of the lens with reference to decentration in or out.

Decentration up or down **(makes/does not make)** any difference whether the lens is right or left, concave side up or toward the graph.

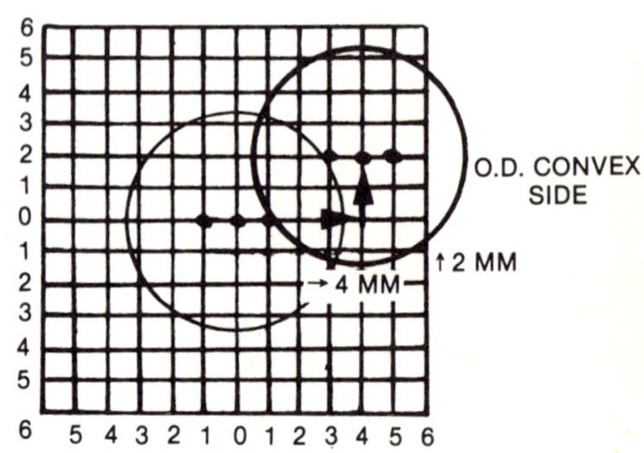

Answer 757. **Go to Frame 758.**

Frame 758. This book, *Volume II: The Science of Opticianry*, is a continuation of the series, *Opticianry: The Practice and the Art: Volume I.*

You will notice that this book begins with frame number **(1/757)**.

Choose the correct response to the multiple choice question and write your answer below.

THEN, TURN TO THE TOP OF PAGE 5, **FRAME 759**

Answer 895. **None required.**

Frame 896. It is not infrequent that decentration is required *both* horizontal and vertical in the same lens. Study the data in this frame. Then calculate the necessary decentration, first horizontally, then vertically.

DATA

P.D.	= 60
A Box	= 52
dbl	= 20
B Box	= 42
O.C. Vertical	= 25

Formulas: Horizontal

$$\frac{(\text{A Box} + \text{dbl}) - (\text{P.D.})}{2} =$$

Vertical

$$\frac{\text{B}}{2} - \text{O.C.} =$$

Answer 1033. None Required

Frame 1034.

CHAPTER 14
ANISOMETROPIA

TURN TO THE TOP OF PAGE 6, **FRAME 1035.**

Answer 1171. Does Not

Frame 1172. It is the decentration in or out that requires the most concentration. It is easy to confuse directions. This Chapter will adopt the plus (convex) side of the lens for decentration reference. Study the illustration in this frame.

In order to correctly place this lens, the Optician decenters to the **(right/left)** and **(up/down)**.

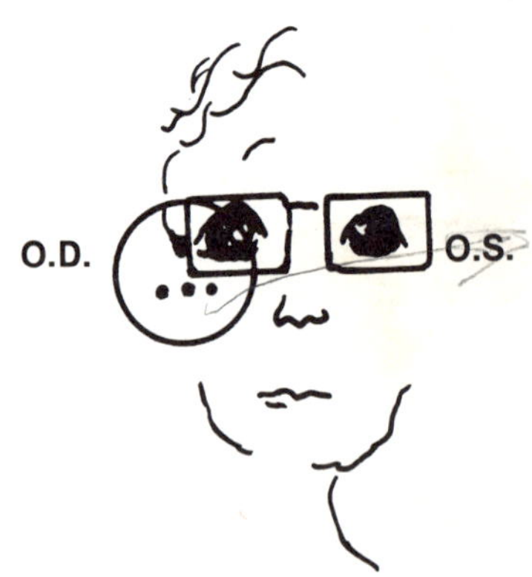

Answer 758. **757**

Frame 759. This book begins with frame number 757, therefore, it would be reasonable to assume that frames numbered 1 thru 756 must be in another volume.

The volume which would logically contain frame numbers 1 thru 756 would be volume **(I/II)**, The Introduction to Dispensing.

Answer 896. **Horizontal = 6** **Vertical = 4**

Frame 897. Since the horizontal frame P.D. (52 + 20 = 72) was greater than the patient's P.D. (60), the decentration would have to be **(inward/outward)**.

Since the vertical geometric center ($\frac{42}{2} = 21$) was lower than the needed O.C. height, (25), the decentration would have to be **(upward/downward)**.

Answer 1034. None Required

Frame 1035. Anisometropia is defined as any difference in lens power between O.D. and O.S. Opticians, however, are mostly concerned with an amount of anisometropia which can result in intolerable prism at the reading level of multifocals.

Intolerable prismatic effect **(is/is not)** of concern to the dispensing Optician.

Answer 1172. Right, Up

Frame 1173. Once the lens is layed out, that is marked for shaping, the working center is affixed to a holding device which inserts into the edger. The holding device rotates, allowing the lens to be shaped against the edging wheel.

The edger "knows" the lens shape from a pattern which must be set in place before the lens is actually shaped. Study the illustration in this frame.

The illustration shows the anatomy of a pattern. The pattern has one large and **(two/three)** small holes.

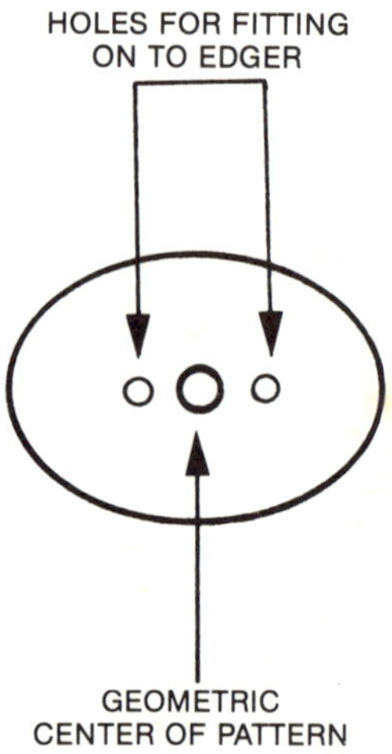

Answer 759. I

Frame 760. Frame numbers 1 thru 756 are in Volume One, Opticianry: The Practice and the Art: Introduction to Dispensing. This volume, Volume II, The Science of Opticianry assumes you already have command of the knowledge learned in the first volume.

Programmed books like this, present a body of information, then a question, which is usually multiple choice. You are then requested to write your answer in the space provided at the bottom of the frame.

Your answer space is at the **(top/bottom).**

Answer 897. inward, upward

Frame 898. The calculation of needed decentration is required by the dispensing Optician for three main reasons: To understand the lab procedure, to determine the needed lens blank size, and to calculate the consequence of decentration itself.

There are **(thirty/three)** main reasons for the Optician to understand the calculation of decentration.

Answer 1035. Is

Frame 1036. The prismatic imbalance is calculated by multiplying the difference between the O.D. and O.S. lens power (in the vertical meridian) times the distance the eyes travel from primary gaze to the reading level.

Study the illustration in this frame. The illustration shows the distance the eyes lower to reading **(level/bevel).**

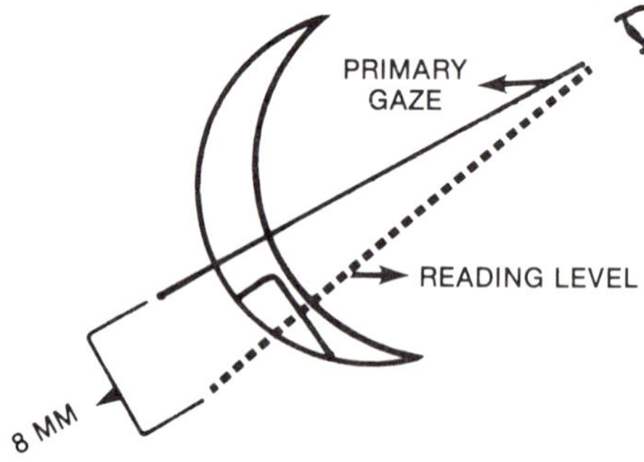

Answer 1173. Two

Frame 1174. As the pattern and lens rotate, the lens is shaped against a grinding stone (diamond wheel) to the pattern shape. Opticians can see the same principle used on key machines where the one key is used as a pattern to make another key.

The ratio between the pattern measurement and a "standard" measurement determines the finished lens size. Since the pattern is rarely the same size as the lens, some compensation will be needed to prevent all sizes from becoming the pattern size!

Pattern sizes **(need/do not need)** to be compensated for.

Answer 760. Bottom

Frame 761. The available space where your answer is to be written is located at the bottom* of the frame. You are requested to write your answer in the space provided and then turn the page to discover the author's answer located at the top of the next frame.

The author's answer is found by turning the page and locating the **(top/bottom)** of the next numerically sequenced frame.

---

*Frame Bottom (your answer space)

Answer 898. Three

Frame 899. Of the three main reasons for the understanding of decentration; the lab procedure of physically moving the optical **(sinner/center)** was discussed in this Chapter, Chapter Eight.

The second reason, that of computing the needed lens blank size, continues in the following Chapter, Chapter Nine.

Turn to Frame 900, Page 11.

Answer 1036. Level

Frame 1037. Multiplying the difference of the vertical lens power (between the two lenses) times the distance from primary gaze to reading level, will equal the prismatic anisometropic effect. Study the Rx in this frame.

O.D. +2.50 +1.50 × 180
O.S. +1.50 +1.00 × 90 ADD +3.00

Reading level 8 mm. below primary gaze.

The total prismatic effect will be
(O.D.+4.00) (−) (O.S.+1.50) = +2.50.

$$\Delta = \frac{d \times P}{10} = \frac{(8)\times(+2.50)}{10} = \frac{20.00}{10}$$

$= 2.0$ **(B.U./B.D.).**

Answer 1174. Need

Frame 1175. The pattern compensation formula is based upon the measurement of 36.5 mm. (which used to be the size of all patterns). The Optician measures the pattern and calculates any difference between it and one which would measure 36.5 mm. Study the example in the frame.

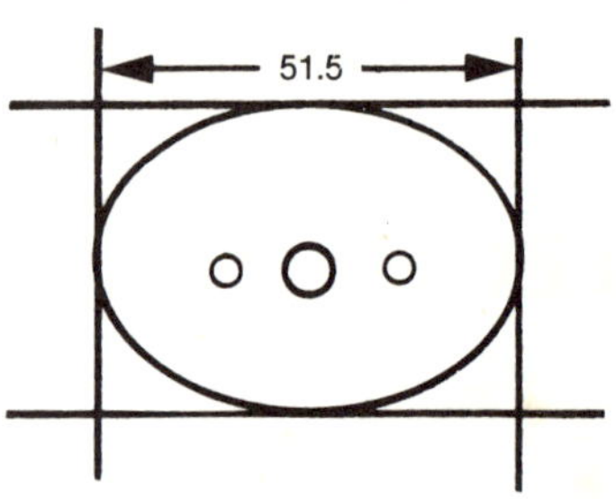

The frame shows the size of the pattern as **(51.5/36.5).**

Answer 761. Top

Frame 762. The author's answer is found at the top of the frame and your written response will be at the bottom of the frame. If your answer was correct, you may move on to the next frame. If your answer differs from the author's answer, you should **(go back and find out why/quit).**

Answer 899. Center

Frame 900.

CHAPTER 9
EFFECTIVE DIAMETER: The Needed Lens Blank Size

TURN TO THE BOTTOM OF PAGE 13, **FRAME 901.**

Answer 1037. B.U.

Frame 1038. When greater than 1.00 D of anisometropia exists at the reading level, the Δ may be compensated in order to be balanced. Study the Rx in this Frame.

O.D. +1.00 −2.00 × 45 ADD +1.50*
O.S. +1.00 −2.00 × 135
Reading level 9 mm. below primary gaze.

This Rx has **(some/no)** prismatic imbalance at reading level.

When computing vertical imbalance, you should disregard the add power.

Answer 1175. 51.5

Frame 1176. The standard for pattern measure ments is 36.5. The pattern in Frame 1175, however, measures 51.5, which means that it is 15 mm. larger than it should have been. If the finished lens size is to be 54 mm., then the Optician subtracts 54 − 15 = 39. So, by setting the edger dial to 39, this finished lens size will become 54 mm.

See if you can reduce this statement to formula form. Then turn to Frame 1177.

F_s = Finished Size
P_s = Pattern Size
E_s = Edger Set

Answer 762. Go back and find out why. If you quit, you'll miss all the fun!

Frame 763. Programmed learning is designed to be easy. That's because it prevents you from going faster than you can learn, so it can be fun.

Programmed learning is **(easy/hard)** and **(boring/fun)**.

Answer 900. None required.

Frame 901. The dispensing Optician needs to know if decentration is possible within a given lens blank size. If decentration is not possible, then extra costs and time may be incurred for the lab to special process extra decentration. The determination of the needed lens blank size is called the E.D. formula.

The determination of E.D. **(can/cannot)** save costs.

Answer 1038. No (Because it is Plano at 90°)

Frame 1039. Test your ability to calculate the imbalances for the following anisometropic Rx's in this frame. Check your answers with the correct solutions in Frame 1040.

Rx	READING LEVEL	AMOUNT OF Δ	DIRECTION OF Δ	IN FRONT OF O.D./O.S.
Example O.D. +4.00 +1.50 × 180 O.S. +3.00 +1.50 × 90 ADD +2.00	8 Below	2 Δ	B.U.	O.D.
A) O.D. +2.00 −2.00 × 45 O.S. +4.00 −4.00 × 135 ADD +1.75	10 Below		?	?
B) O.D. −6.00 Sph O.S. −2.00 Sph ADD +2.75	9 Below		?	?
C) O.D. +1.00 Sph O.S. +4.00 Sph ADD +2.00	7 Below		?	?
D) O.D. Plano −4.00 × 120 O.S. −3.00 −1.00 × 180 ADD +2.75	8 Below		?	?

Answer 1176. $\mathbf{E_s = F_s - (P_s - 36.5)}$

Frame 1177. See if your formula works. Here is the data.

Finished Lens Size (F_s) = 54 mm
Pattern Size (P_s) = 51.5
Edger Set (E_s) = ?

$$E_s = F_s - (P_s - 36.5)$$
$$E_s = 5.4 - (51.5 - 36.5)$$
$$E_s = 5.4 - 15$$
$$E_s = 39$$

When the pattern size is smaller than 36.5, then the difference must be **(added/divided)**.

Answer 763. Easy, fun

Frame 764. Now either choose a Chapter of interest from the Table of Contents or turn the page to Frame 765 and begin.*

Enjoy!

*Remember, though, the material presented is accumulative and builds upon what has been learned before. Therefore, accumulating the knowledge in this book as it is designed, chapter by chapter, allows for your greatest chances for success in learning.

Answer 901. Can

Frame 902. E.D. are the initials for Effective Diameter. The E.D. plus **2 times** the decentration will yield the needed lens blank size. The E.D. is defined as twice the distance from the geometric center of the lens, to its furthest edge.

Study the illustration in this frame. Twice line **(A – C/C – B)** best illustrates the E.D.

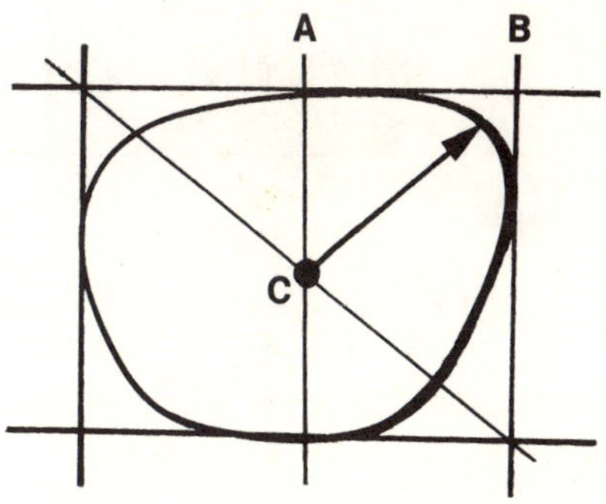

Answer 1039. **See below. (If you missed any of these, you may need to review Chapter Thirteen.)**

Frame 1040.

P	×	d	=		÷	10	=	Δ		
DIFFERENCE IN VERTICAL MERIDIAN	×	READING DEPTH	=		÷		=	Δ	BASE	O.D./O.S.
A) +1.00	×	10	=	10	÷	10	=	1.0	B.U.	O.S.
B) −4.00	×	9	=	36	÷	10	=	3.6	B.D.	O.D.
C) +3.00	×	7	=	21	÷	10	=	2.1	B.U.	O.S.
D) −3.00	×	8	=	24	÷	10	=	2.4	B.D.	O.S.

The Rx's most needing the Optician's attention are **(AC/BD).**

____

Answer 1177. **Added**

Frame 1178. Test your skill at determining the correct edger setting from the data below.

	F_s WHEN FINISHED LENS SIZE IS	−	(P_s) AND PATTERN MEASURES	+ −	(36.5) ADD OR SUBTRACT	= TO GET	E_s EDGER SET
Example:	56	−	(41.5)	−	(36.5)	=	51
A)	55	−	(46.5)	?		=	?
B)	53	−	(48.0)	?		=	?
C)	50	−	(36.5)	?		=	?
D)	51.5	−	(51.5)	?		=	?
E)	48	−	(51)	?		=	?

____

Answer 764. None required.

Frame 765.

CHAPTER 2
THE Rx ANALYSIS

PLEASE TURN TO **FRAME 766**, ON THE TOP OF PAGE 19

Answer 902. C-B

Frame 903. The effective diameter is calculated as: twice the radius from the geometric center of the lens to its furthest edge. If the radius is 35, then the E.D. is said to be twice 35 or 70. The dispenser can calculate the E.D. by measuring the longest frame diameter with a millimeter rule.

Study the illustration in this frame. The E.D. is best illustrated by example **(A/B).**

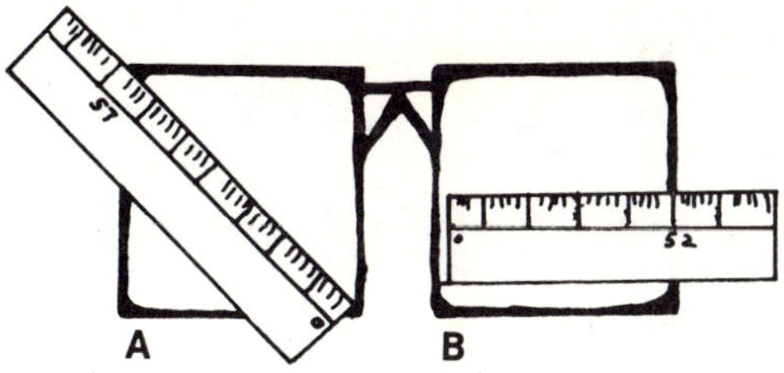

Answer 1040. B, D (That was a taxing frame!)

Frame 1041. The Optician is able to compensate for vertical imbalance in one of five ways. The first way avoids the problems of anisometropia by eliminating the need for the bifocal.

The patient still requires lenses for distance **and** reading, thus, a separate pair for distance and a separate pair for **(reading/intermediate)** glasses solves the problem.

____

Answer 1178. A) 45, B) 41.5, C) 50, D) 36.5 E) 33.5

Frame 1179. When layout involves multifocals, the Optician uses the seg line as a reference point for vertical decentration. If more than one seg line is present, as in trifocals, the Optician references the top line. Study the problem in this frame.

A) O.D. Rx = +2.00 +4.00 x 180
ADD +2.50
B) Seg Height = 22
C) 'A' Box = 55
D) 'B' Box = 46
E) Dbl = 18
F) P.D. = 64/61

How many mm. must the seg be decentered vertically?

The Optician needs **(all/only some)** of the data.

____

Answer 765. No answer needed.

Frame 766. The Optician analyzes the doctor's prescription to determine its meaning. The Rx tells the Optician two things: first, the nature of the ametropia and second, the profile of the needed lens.

Rx analysis reveals the nature of the ametropia and the lens **(profile/argyle).**

Answer 903. A

Frame 904. The needed lens blank size diameter is defined as the E.D. plus 2 times the monocular decentration. Study the data in the example in this frame. The needed lens blank size equals the E.D. plus one-half of ('A' Box + dbl) - (PD).

Example: **DATA**

'A' Box = 54
P.D. = 62
dbl = 18
E.D. = 56

Here is how it works:

$$NLBS = ED + \frac{(\text{'A' Box} + dbl) - (P.D.)}{2}$$

$$NLBS = 56 + \frac{(54+18) - (62)}{2}$$

$$NLBS = 56 + \frac{(72) - (62)}{2}$$

$$NLBS = 56 + \frac{10}{2}$$

$$NLBS = 56 + 5$$

$$NLBS = 61$$

The needed lens blank is **(16/61).**

Answer 1041. Reading.

Frame 1042. Separate glasses for distance and reading are the first method of compensating for anisometropia. Study the Rx in this frame.

O.D. +3.00 +2.00 × 180 ADD +2.00
O.S. +2.00 +1.75 × 90
Reading level 8 Below

Ths prismatic imbalance of this Rx is **(2.4 B.U./ 2.4 B.D.)** at 8 mm. below for reading.

The Optician may use **(One/Two)** pairs of glasses to solve the anisometropia.

Answer 1179. Only some.

Frame 1180. The data which concerns vertical decentration is: seg height and 'B' Box only. In the last frame, those were:

Seg Height = 22
'B' Box = 46

Calculate the Vertical Decentration (V_d)

$$V_d = \frac{\text{'B' Box}}{2}^{*} - \text{Seg Height}$$

$$V_d = \frac{46}{2} - 22$$

$$V_d = 23 - 22$$

V_d = 1 mm. **(Up/Down)**

Note: If Seg Height is greater than $\frac{\text{'B' Box}}{2}$, then decentration is up. If Seg Height is less than $\frac{\text{'B' Box}}{2}$, then decentration will be down.

Answer 766. profile

Frame 767. The Rx +1.00 +2.00 x 180 says to the Optician, "I am a prescription for ametropia composed of plus one diopter of power for the correction of **(myopia/hyperopia),**" and "I am also combined with **(+1.00/+2.00)** diopters of power for the correction of astigmatism.

Answer 904. 61

Frame 905. E.D. deals with cutting out a given lens shape, including decentration, from the smallest possible circle of lens material. Unfortunately, the E.D. formula is theoretical and does not take the lens edge into consideration.

The E.D. formula **(does/does not)** take into account the lens edge.

Answer 1042. 2.4 B.U., Two

Frame 1043. Which two sets of Rx's below solve the problem in Frame 1042?

A) O.D. +5.00 +2.00 x 180
O.S. +4.00 +1.75 x 90

B) O.D. +3.00 +2.00 x 180
O.S. +2.00 +1.75 x 90

C) O.D. +2.00 +2.00 x 180
O.S. +4.00 +2.00 x 90 2.4 B.U.

D) O.D. +5.00 +2.00 x 180 2.0 B.D.
O.S. +4.00 +1.75 x 90 2.0 B.U.

Answer 1180. Down

Frame 1181. Study the examples of multifocals in this frame, and determine 1) the amount of vertical decentration required and, 2) the direction the Optician must move the seg line.

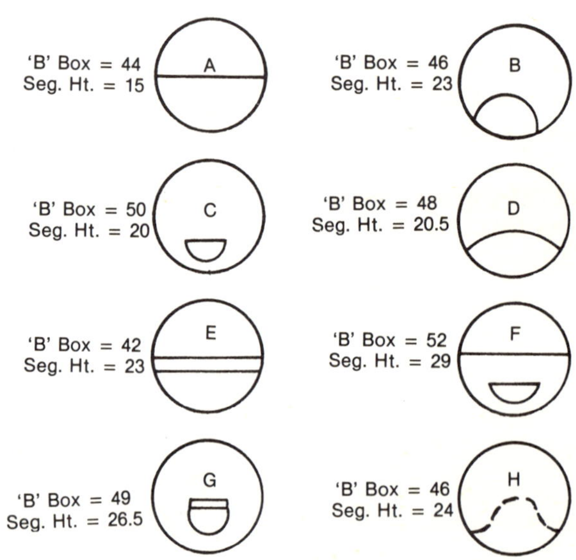

Answer 767. Hyperopia, +2.00

Frame 768. Study the example in this frame.

The example shows the Rx as it is intended to be read; that is, plus one sphere combined with a +2.00 cylinder whose axis is 180 degrees.

(+1.00) (+2.00 x 180)

or

+1.00 ⊙ +2.00 x 180

What the Rx +1.00 +2.00 x 180 really says to the optician is "I am a prescription of +1.00 sphere combined with a cylinder of +2.00 whose axis is **(180/090).**"

Answer 905. does not

Frame 906. Most lenses do not carry the prescription all the way to the very edge. This is especially true with molded or cast blanks. In addition, there is frequently lens edge treatment to be performed such as beveling for the frame groove.

Because the Optician needs extra room at the edge, the E.D. formula really **(should/should not)** be modified to allow sufficient edge room.

Answer 1043. A and B

Frame 1044. Two separate pairs of glasses is the first of five ways the Optician can solve problems of anisometropia. The second choice for compensating anisometropic Rx's is by the use of dissimilar segments.

Study the example in this frame.

The example shows **(similar/dissimilar)** segments.

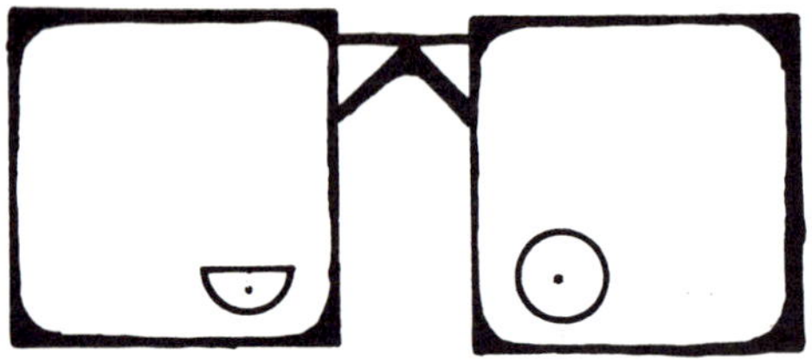

____

Answer 1181. **A) 7 down - B) on center - C) 5 down - D) 3.5 down - E) 2 up - F) 3 up - G) 2 up - H) 1 up**

Frame 1182. This Chapter on Cutting and Edging involves multiple procedures, so, lets stop a moment and get control of it all . . . remember, this book is supposed to make things easy and fun.

Now, relax, go ahead, close your eyes, and count backward from +10.00 (in Diopters).

While you're doing so, memorize Ashkenazi's famous rule of cutting and edging: Measure twice, cut once.

____

Answer 768. 180, of course.

Frame 769. By separating the sphere, from the cylinder and its axis, the Optician can mentally visualize the prescription as a combination of two optical graphs.

Study the illustration in this frame. The sphere is represented by graph **(A/B)** and the cylinder is represented as **(B/A).**

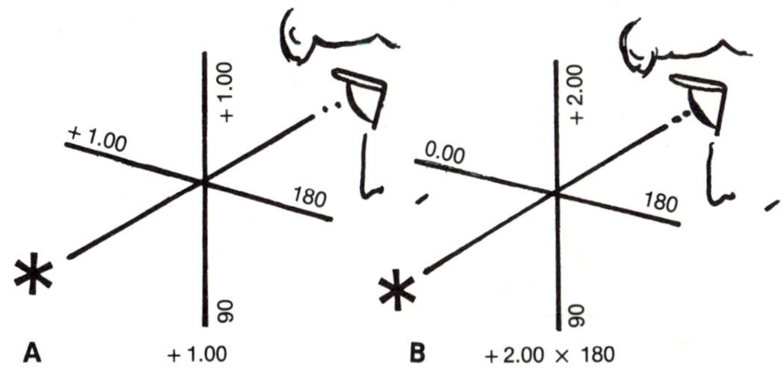

Answer 906. should

Frame 906. Consider the E.D. formula once again. This time from memory. (NLBS) Needed lens blank size = the lens E.D. + **(monocular/-binocular)** decentration.

Answer 1044. Dissimilar.

Frame 1045. One formula for calculating the needed dissimilar segment is:

$$ds = \frac{r\ (vp+A)}{A}$$ Where

ds = dissimilar seg
r = reading level
A = Add Power
vp = Vertical Power

Study the Rx and needed data in this frame.

O.D. +3.00 +1.00 × 90
O.S. +0.75 +2.00 × 90 ADD +3.00
Reading level 11 Below. Seg 3 below distance O.C.

The anisometropia (vertical imbalance) is **(2.5/5.2) (B.U./B.D.)**.

Answer 1182. None required, that was a rest frame.

Frame 1183. Let's use the pause for a summary:

1) Cutting and Edging is really laying out for decentration, and then shaping.

2) Layout is performed on a grid and may include both horizontal as well as vertical decentration.

3) Horizontal decentration for each eye is calculated by the formula:

$$H_d = \frac{(\text{'A' Box}+\text{dbl}) - (\text{P.D.})}{2}$$

4) Vertical decentration is calculated by the formula $V_d = \frac{\text{'B' Box}}{2} - \text{O.C. or Seg ht.}$

5) Patterns are referenced at 36.5.

6) Edger set formula = finished lens size − (pattern size − 36.5).

Because it is crucial that the Optician keep track of left and right, it would be wise to mark the lens with a grease pencil to **(prevent/encourage)** mix-ups.

Answer 769. **A, B.**

Frame 770. The *combined* graphs, or optical crosses, form the second portion of the Rx analysis: The Lens Profile.

Study the illustration in this frame. The illustration shows how the power is distributed throughout the needed lens.

This lens has +1.00 diopters of power in the 180° meridian and **(+2.00/+3.00)** diopters of power in the 90° meridian.

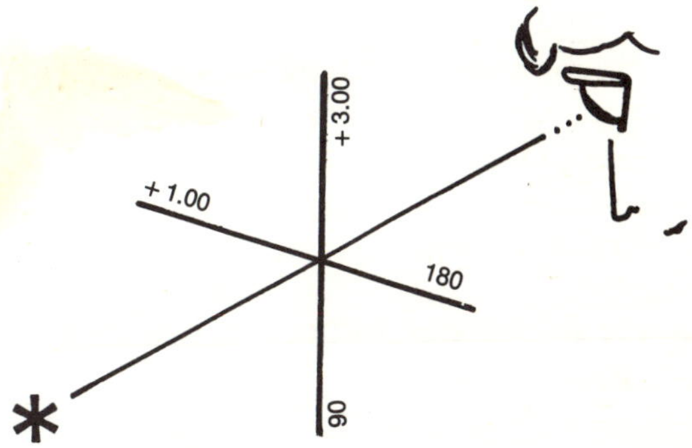

Answer 907. **Binocular**

Frame 908. The needed lens blank size = E.D. -+ monocular decentration times 2. The monocular decentration, as you will remember, is

$$\frac{(\text{'A' Box} + \text{dbl} - \text{P.D.})}{2} . \quad \frac{(\text{'A' Box} + \text{dbl} - \text{P.D.})}{2}$$

+ (E.D.) = Needed Lens Blank Size.

Study the two formulas below. The formula which would allow for the largest amount of room would be that formula which provides for extra decentration **(A/B)**.

N.L.B.S. =

A

$$(\text{'A' Box} + \text{dbl}) - (\text{P.D.}) + \text{E.D.}$$

B

$$\frac{(\text{'A' Box} + \text{dbl} - \text{P.D.})}{2} + \text{E.D.}$$

Answer 1045. 2.5, B.U.

Frame 1046. Continue with the dissimilar segment formula in Frame 1045:

$$\text{O.D. ds} = \frac{r\ (vp+A)}{A} = \frac{11\ (3.00+3.00)}{3.00} = 22$$

ds = 22 . . .   **BUT . . .**

The segs are already 3 Below distance O.C., **SO:** 22 − 3 = 19. The distance needed from the seg top to its O.C. is 19 mm. Study the bifocals in this frame. The style with its O.C. 19 mm. from the top is **(A/B/C).**

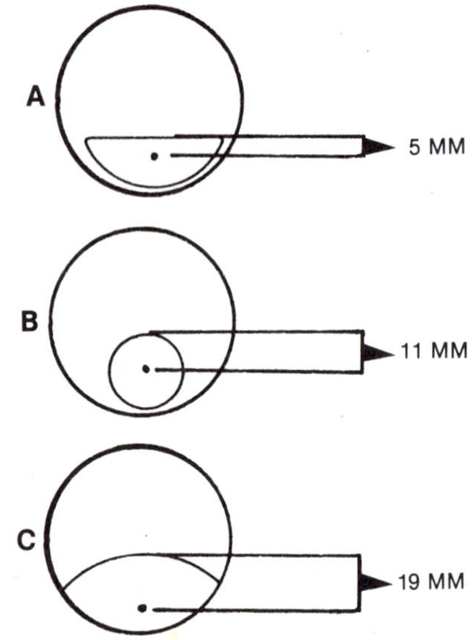

Answer 1183. Prevent.

Frame 1184. When layout is performed for multifocals, the seg line is used as a vertical reference. Horizontal decentration, for P.D., however, must use the near P.D. reading. That's important!

Because the eyes converge when they are lowered to read, the P.D. for the distance and the P.D. for near or reading **(cannot/can)** be the same.

Answer 770. **+3.00.**

Frame 771. Understanding the lens profile enables the Optician to better guide the patient to proper frame selection. The Optician must be able to visualize the finished lens product in order to best select the most appropriate frame to surround the lens.

Rx mental visualization helps to understand the **(lens/frame)** profile.

Answer 908. **A.**

Frame 909. The 'A' Box +dbl can be called the Frame P.D. or F.P.D. The formula then becomes N.L.B.S. = E.D. + (F.P.D. − P.P.D.)

Where: N.L.B.S. = Needed Lens Blank Size
F.P.D. = Frame P.D. ('A' Box+dbl)
P.P.D. = Patient's P.D.
E.D. = Effective Diameter of lens.

If F.P.D. = 74, P.P.D. = 64, and E.D. = 58, then N.L.B.S. would = **(68/78)**.

Answer 1046. C.

Frame 1047. An ultex style has its O.C. 19 mm. from the seg top. Continue with the original Rx in Frame 1045 . . .

$$\text{O.S. ds} = \frac{r\,(vp+A)}{A} = \frac{11\,(0.75 + 3.00)}{3.00} = 14 \text{ mm.}$$

14 − 3 = 11 mm.

The needed bifocal style is one in which the distance from the seg top to its O.C. is 11 mm. from the three examples in Frame 1046, that style is **(A/B/C).**

Answer 1184. Cannot.

Frame 1185. The P.D. for near is used for horizontal decentration calculation of multifocals. Study the Rx and Data in this frame. The near P.D. is **(64/61).**

Rx	= −3.75 − 0.75 × 135 / Add +2.50
P.D.	= 64 / 61
E.D.	= 68
'A' Box	= 62
'B' Box	= 54
Seg ht	= 23
Dbl	= 18

The Optician uses the near P.D. for calculating the total horizontal decentration. Which do you think is the correct formula: **(A/B)**?

A) Decentration = (62+18) − 64
B) Decentration = (62+18) − 61

Answer 771. Lens

Frame 772. The Optician mentally visualizes the lens as it sits in front of the patient's eye.

Study the illustration in this frame. The illustration shows an eye looking down a visual line of sight. The eye is the **(patient's/optician's).**

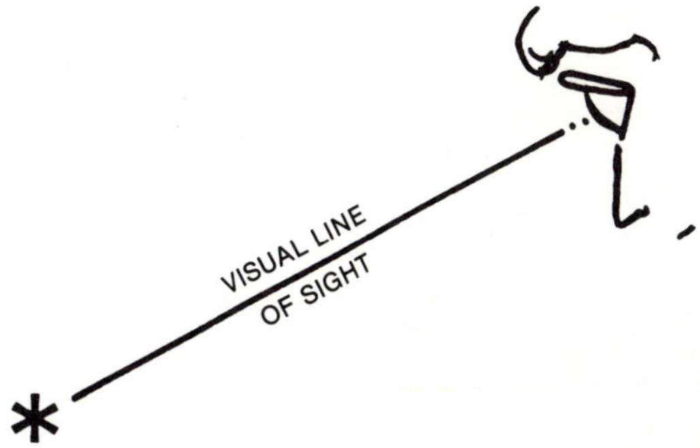

Answer 909. 68

Frame 910. E.D. plus total decentration will more than provide the Optician with a needed lens blank size guide which will provide for sufficient edge room. However, dependent upon prescription and lens shape, a smaller diameter may sometimes be used.

The dispensing Optician should use the author's formula for N.L.B.S. as a **(absolute/recommended)** guideline.

Answer 1047. B.

Frame 1048. The Optician can balance the anisometropia of 2.4 B.U. in the Rx:

O.D. +3.00 +1.00 × 90 ADD +3.00
O.S. +0.75 +2.00 × 90

Reading level 11 Below. Seg tops 3 Below dist O.C. with O.D. **(A/B)** and O.S. **(A/B)**.

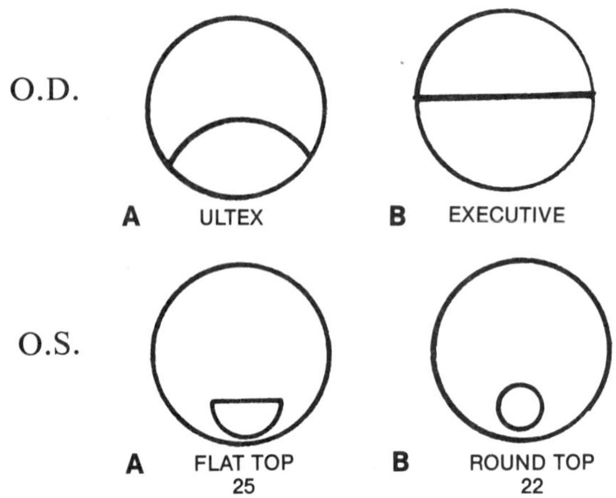

Answer 1185. 61, B.

Frame 1186. The near P.D. is to be used when Opticians lay out multifocals for horizontal decentration. Study the example in this frame.

Rx O.D. −0.50 +1.50 × 165 ADD +2.25
O.S. −0.75 +2.00 × 75

P.D. = 63/60
'A' Box = 54
'B' Box = 44
Dbl = 18
Seg ht = 18

Horizontal decentration $= \frac{(54+18) - (60)}{2}$

= 6 mm. each.
The lens must be decentered 6 mm. **(in/out)**.

Answer 772. Patients'

Frame 773. With a mental picture of the Patient's eye sighting along a visual line of sight, the Optician can now graph the prescription in front of the eye.

Mentally place the prescription −2.00 +1.00 × 180 on the visual line of sight provided in this frame. Check your answer in Frame 774.

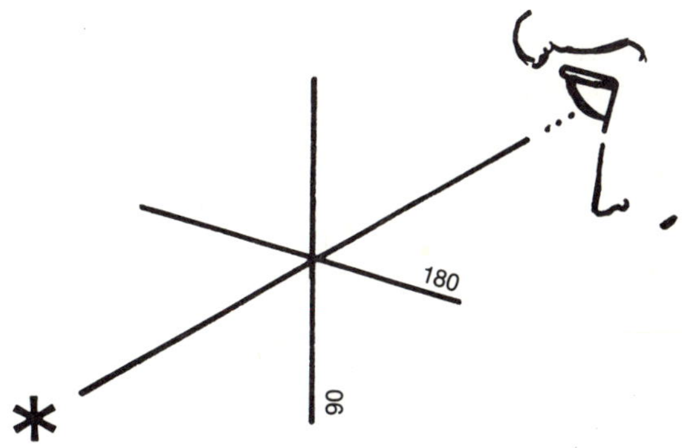

Answer 910. Recommended.

Frame 911. Test your skill at estimating the N.L.B.S. for the following lenses from the chart below.

	F.P.D. ('A' Box+dbl)		P.P.D.	E.D.	N.L.B.S.
Example:	52	20	60	56	68
A)	54	18	63	57	?
B)	56	16	61	59	?
C)	50	18	69	50	?
D)	53	17	56	55	?

Answer 1048. O.D. A, O.S. B.

Frame 1049. Actually, lots of imbalance can be compensated for by using dissimilar segments. Study the Rx and data in this frame.

O.D. −1.00 sph 22 Round Top seg (O.C. 11 Below)
O.S. −4.00 sph 22 Flat Top seg (O.C. 4 Below)
ADD +2.00
Reading level 8 Below.

O.D. $\Delta = \frac{d \times P}{10} = \frac{8 \times 1}{10} = 0.8$ B.D.

The calculation illustrated is for the **(distance/near)** prismatic effect.

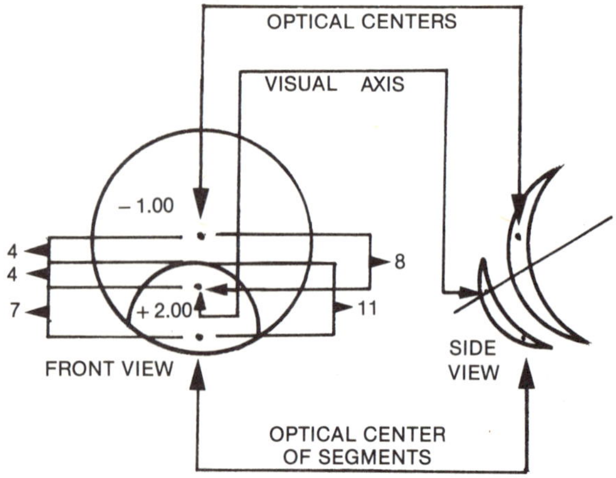

Answer 1186. In.

Frame 1187. When layout includes a prescription with prism, the Optician must coordinate knowledge of both horizontal and vertical decentration, prism, E.D., cylinder analysis, P.D. and patterns. Study the problem in this frame.

DATA O.D. = +4.00 sph 2 B.I.
P.D. = 62
'A' Box = 51
'B' Box = 41
Dbl = 17

Question: How much decentration and in what direction will this Rx have to be decentered?

The question is in **(one/two)** parts.

Answer 773. Go to frame 774.

Frame 774. Your answer should look like this:

The Rx −200 +1.00 x 180 has **(−1.00/−2.00)** diopters of power at its axis.

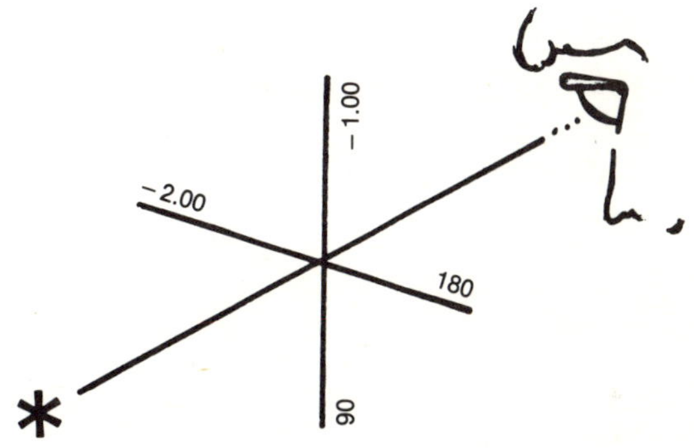

Answer 911. A = 66, B = 70, C = 51, D = 69

Frame 912. If the N.L.B.S. is equal to or less than the available lens diameter, then the decentration and shaping may be accomplished. If the N.L.B.S. is greater than the available lens diameter, then decentration may **not** be accomplished and the lens will need additional **(processing/be impossible).**

Additional processing may include placing the decentration **within** the lens blank and will be discussed in another chapter.

Answer 1049. Distance.

Frame 1050. Continue with the calculation once again. This frame reproduces the O.D. lens in Frame 1049. The distance prismatic calculation is:

$$\Delta = \frac{d \times P}{10} = \frac{8 \times (-1.00)}{10} = 0.8 \text{ B.D.}$$

The reading calculation is:

$$\Delta = \frac{d \times P}{10} = \frac{7 \times (+2.00)}{10} = 1.4 \text{ B.D.}$$

The combined prismatic effect of the distance and near is calculated as:

0.8 B.D. (distance)
+ 1.4 B.D. (reading)
2.2 B.D.

Now, turn to Frame 1051 and calculate the **(O.S./O.U.)**.

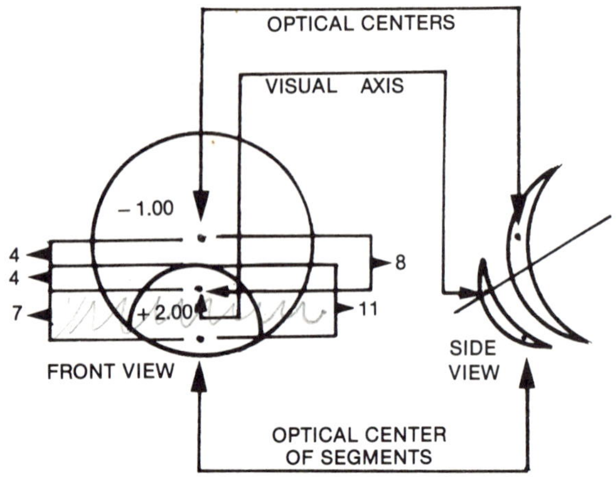

Answer 1187. Two.

Frame 1188.

Part One: A How much does the lens need to be decentered for P.D.?

B How much does the lens need to be decentered for Δ?

A. $\frac{(51+17)-(62)}{2} = 3$ mm.

B. $d = \frac{10\Delta}{P} = \frac{10 \times 2\Delta}{+4.00} = \frac{20}{+4.00}$

$= 5$ mm.

Part Two: In what direction?

A Frame P.D. is larger than Patient's P.D., therefore, decenter in 3 mm.

B Plus lenses are decentered in for Δ B.I., therefore, decenter in 5 mm.

The total decentration required to create Δ 2 B.I., for +4.00 sph with a 62 P.D., therefore, must be **(2/8)**.

Answer 774. **−2.00**

Frame 775. The illustration in frame 774 shows how the power is distributed in a lens of −2.00 +1.00 x 180.

Test your mastery of mental visualization of an Rx by correctly placing the following prescriptions on the visual lines of sight provided in this frame. Your answers should coincide with those in frame 776.

A) −4.00 +2.00 x 090
B) +1.00 −3.00 x 180
C) −2.50 −2.50 x 090
D) +3.75 +0.75 x 180

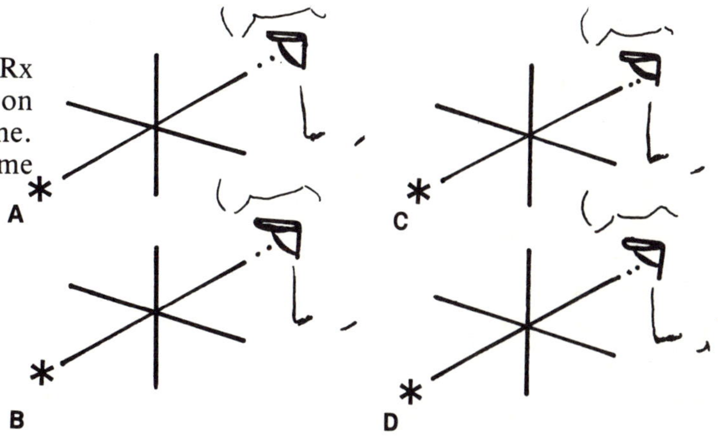

Answer 912. **processing.**

Frame 913. Back in Chapter Eight, Frame Nos. 898, 899, mentioned three main reasons for the Optician to fully understand decentration:

1) To understand the lab procedure.
2) To determine the needed lens blank size.
3) To calculate the consequence of the decentration process, (prism).

This chapter dealt with **(1/2/3)** of the above.

Answer 1050. O.S.

Frame 1051. The O.S. Rx −4.00 Sph. ADD +2.00. Notice that the O.S. illustrated is a flat top. Using the same technique as with O.D., calculate the combined prismatic effect of the distance and near $\Delta = \frac{d \times P}{10} = \frac{(8) \times (-4.00)}{10} = \frac{32}{10} = 3.2$ B.D.

At 8 mm. below the distance optical center, the visual line of sight passes directly through the seg **(center/edge)**.

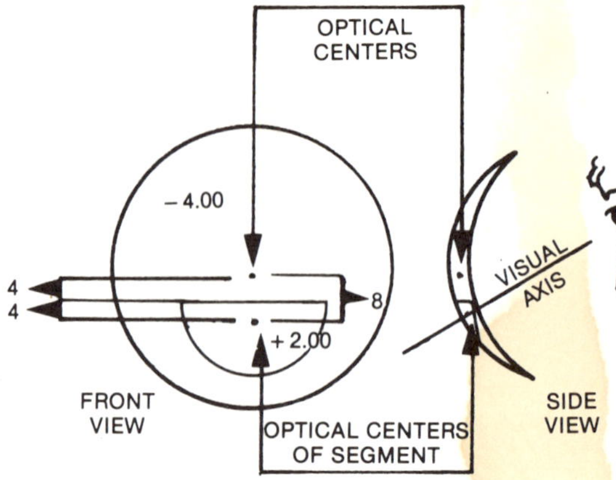

Answer 1188. 8.

Frame 1189. Try another one.

DATA Rx = O.D. −2.50 sph 3 Δ B.I.
O.S. −3.50 sph 3 Δ B.I.
P.D. = 62
'A' Box = 56
'B' Box = 49
Dbl = 18

Question: How much total decentration and in what direction is required to layout these two lenses for edging?

Are you ready? **(Yes/No)**

Answer 775. Go to Frame 776.

Frame 776. These Rx's as pictured are only **(one/two)** dimensional.

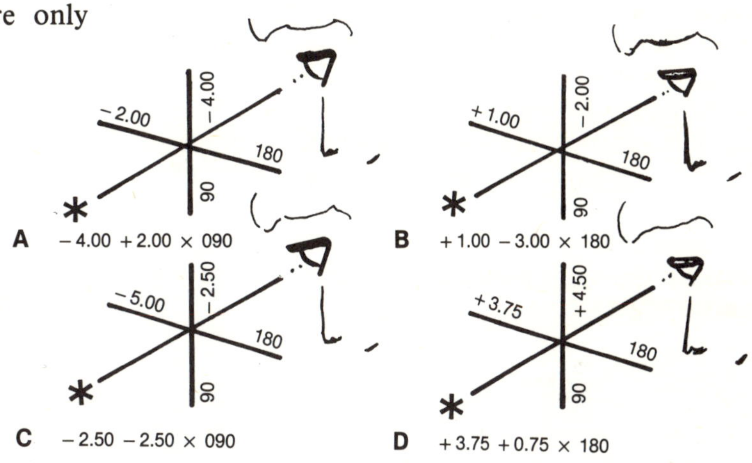

Answer 913. **2**

Frame 914.

CHAPTER 10
THE CONSEQUENCE OF DECENTRATION: PRISM

PLEASE TURN TO THE
BOTTOM OF PAGE 41, **FRAME 915.**

Answer 1051. Center

Frame 1052. At 8 mm. below the distance O.C., the visual line of sight passes exactly through the segment's O.C.

When the visual line of sight passes exactly through the O.C. of any lens, the prism created is **(0/180)**.

Answer 1189. Yes. (Opticians aren't chickens.)

Frame 1190.

O.D. A. Decentration for P.D.
B. Decentration for △.

A. $\frac{(56+18) - (62)}{2} = 6$ mm. in

B. $d = \frac{10 \times \Delta}{P} = \frac{10 \times 3}{-2.50} = \frac{30}{-2.50}$

$= 12$ mm. out

Therefore, total decentration of 6 in + 12 out = 6 mm. out.

O.S. A. Decentration for P.D.
B. Decentration for △

A. $\frac{(56+18) - (62)}{2} = 6$ mm. in

B. $d = \frac{10 \times \Delta}{P} = \frac{10 \times 3}{-3.50} = \frac{30}{-3.50}$

$= 8.5$ mm. out

Therefore, total decentration of 6 in + 8.5 out = 2.5 mm. out.

The Optician decenters the O.D. 6 mm. out and the O.S. 2.5 mm. out to achieve 3 △ B.I. each eye and total P.D. of **(62/64)**.

Answer 776. one

Frame 777. The Rx's pictured in frame 776 are only one dimensional. However, they accurately depict how the power is distributed throughout the lens.

In order to fully visualize the finished product, the Optician must now add dimension to the visual image.

The visual image, to be realistic, requires **(dimension/diminuation).**

Answer 914. none required

Frame 915. The third main reason for the Optician to understand decentration is its consequence: PRISM.

Prism **(is/is not)** a consequence of decentration.

Answer 1052. Zero. You've got it!

Frame 1053. The correct calculation for the O.S. near only is $\Delta = \frac{d \times P}{10} = \frac{(0) \times (+2.00)}{10} = 0$.

You will recall that the distance prism was 3.2 B.D. 3.2 B.D. plus 0 = 3.2 B.D.

To summarize, the combined prismatic effect of O.D. 2.2^{Δ}B.D. and O.S. 3.2^{Δ}B.D. equals 1.0^{Δ}B.D. Since the Δ is greater before the O.S., the Optician knows the prismatic effect is 1^{Δ}B.D. **(O.D./O.S.)**.

Answer 1190. 62.

Frame 1191. When compound Rx's have axis other than 180, the layout Optician must calculate the total power in the meridian in question. Look at the problem and solution in this frame.

DATA: Rx O.D. −4.00 +2.00 × 90 2^{Δ}B.I.
O.S. Plano +4.00 × 45 1^{Δ}B.O.
P.D. = 64
'A' Box = 55
'B' Box = 46
Dbl = 19

Question: What is the layout decentration for each eye? This time, work your own answers and compare with the solution in the next frame.

Answer 777. Dimension.

Frame 778. Dimension of the mental visual picture is added using base curves, lens material, thickness, size and decentration.

The Optician adds dimension to the lens graph by designing the lens. The tools used are base curve, lens material (index of refraction), size, thickness and **(decentration/decentralization)**.

Answer 915. Is.

Frame 916. Prism is a consequence of decentration. If prism is wanted, then it may be called positive prism. If prism is unwanted, then it may be called **(negative/neutral)** prism.

Answer 1053. O.S.

Frame 1054. Refer back to the original Rx in Frame 1049. If both seg styles were the same, the vertical imbalance would have been Δ 2.4 B.D. However, with dissimilar segs, the Δ has been reduced to a mere Δ 1.0 B.D.

Want to try another one? **(Yes/No)**

Answer 1191. Go to Frame 1192.

Frame 1192.

O.D. A. Decentration for P.D.
B. Decentration for Δ.

A. $\frac{(55+19)-(64)}{2} = 5$ in

B. $d = \frac{10 \times \Delta}{P} = \frac{10 \times 2}{-2.00} = 10$ mm. out

Total = 5 in + 10 out = 5 mm. out

O.S. A. Decentration for P.D.
B. Decentration for Δ.

A. $\frac{(55+19)-(64)}{2} = 5$ in

B. $d = \frac{10 \times \Delta}{P} = \frac{10 \times 1}{+2.00} = \frac{10}{+2.00}$

$= 5$ mm. out

Total = 5 in + 5 out = 0 Decentration!

Sometimes lay out **(requires/never requires)** zero decentration.

Answer 778. Decentration.

Frame 779. The Optician begins designing the lens by choosing base curves, lens material, size and decentration, all of which **(can/cannot)** affect the finished product.

Answer 916. Negative.

Frame 917. Decentering (moving the O.C.) in or out, up or down, to coincide with the line of sight **(creates/negates)** prism.

Because this decentration is necessary and required, the subsequent prism may be called **(positive/negative)**.

Answer 1054. Yes, I knew you were hooked!

. . . .

Frame 1055. Please study the Rx and data in this frame:

O.D. −2.00 ULTEX A
O.S. −9.00 FLAT TOP ADD +3.00
Reading Level 8 Below

Calculate the vertical imbalance for each lens, first for the distance, then for the Add. Then check your answers with the correct one in Frame 1056.

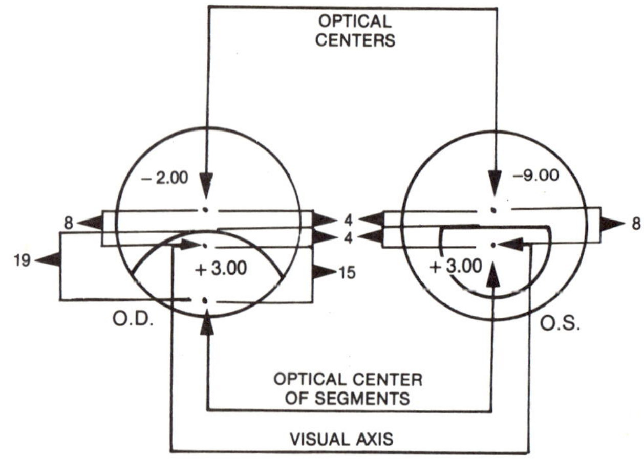

Answer 1192. Requires.

. . . .

Frame 1193. Naturally, when decentration to achieve P.D. and/or prism exceeds the lens blank size, the lab must grind prism into the lens. Test your skill at layout by completing the chart below. Check your answers in the next frame.

Rx	Δ	'A' Box	'B' Box	Dbl	P.D.	=	Total Decentration + Direction
Ex: −2.00 sph	2^{Δ}B. I.	54	44	20	64	=	5 mm. out
A) +3.00 + 2.00 × 90	2^{Δ}B. I.	53	41	16	62	=	?
B) −6.00 − 1.00 × 45	3^{Δ}B.O.	52	42	18	66	=	?
C) +4.00 − 2.00 × 180	4^{Δ}B.O.	55	43	20	69	=	?
D) −5.00 + 3.00 × 135	2.5^{Δ}B. I.	51	40	19	65	=	?

Answer 779. Can.

Frame 780.

CHAPTER 3
LENS DESIGN

TURN TO **FRAME 781** ON THE TOP OF PAGE 49.

Answer 917. Creates, positive.

Frame 918. Decentering to achieve P.D. is considered creating positive prism. Failure to decenter, then, creates negative **(prision/prism)**.

Answer 1055. See below.

Frame 1056.

Distance: $\Delta = \frac{d \times P}{10} = \frac{(8)\times(-2.00)}{10} = 1.6 \text{ B.D.}$

Add: $\Delta = \frac{d \times P}{10} = \frac{(15)\times(+3.00)}{10} = 4.5 \text{ B.D.}$

TOTAL: 6.1 B.D.

Distance: $\Delta = \frac{d \times P}{10} = \frac{(8)\times(-9.00)}{10} = 7.2 \text{ B.D.}$

Add: $\Delta = \frac{d \times P}{10} = \frac{(0)\times(+3.00)}{10} = 0$

TOTAL: 7.2 B.D.

When similar Δ (B.U. and B.U. OR B.D. and B.D.) exists in the same lens, the total is the sum of the two. When similar prism exists in different lenses as in this example of O.D. and O.S., then the total is the difference of the two.

The net prismatic effect for this Rx is **(13.2 B.D./ 1.1 B.D.)**.

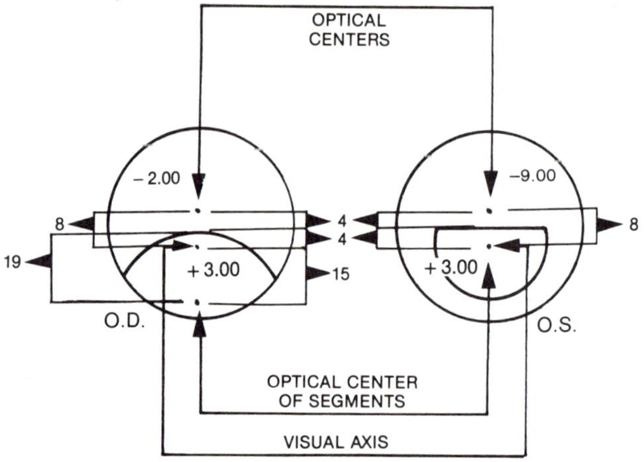

Answer 1193. See Below.

Frame 1194.

Rx	Δ	'A' Box	'B' Box	Dbl	P.D.	=	Total To Be Decentered
A) +3.00 + 2.00 × 90	2^{Δ}B. I.	53	41	16	62	=	7.5 in
B) −6.00 − 1.00 × 45	3^{Δ}B.O.	52	42	18	66	=	6.6 in
C) +4.00 − 2.00 × 180	4^{Δ}B.O.	55	43	20	69	=	7.0 out
D) −5.00 + 3.00 × 135	2.5^{Δ}B. I.	51	40	19	65	=	4.6 out

When prism vertical is asked for, the Optician must calculate horizontal (for P.D.) as well as **(oblique/ vertical)** decentration.

*The Optician may round off for practical layout.

Answer 780. No response needed.

Frame 781. The Optician begins to design the lens by choosing how the lens will be made.

Lens design begins with how the lens will be **(maid/made)**.

Answer 918. Prism.

Frame 919. Just exactly how much prism is created or left out depends upon two factors:

1. The amount of decentration, and
2. The power of the lens.

There are **(too/two)** factors used to calculate the amount of prism.

Answer 1056. 1.1 B.D.

Frame 1057. If the seg styles in Frame 1056 were both the same, then the anisometropia at a point 8 mm. below the distance O.C. would have been 5.6 **(B.U./B.D.)**. By using dissimilar segments, the Optician was able to reduce the imbalance to 1.1 B.D.

There are four ways for the Optician to combat anisometropia in multifocals. The first is **(two/three)** separate pairs, the second is non-**(similar/familiar)** segs.

Answer 1194. Vertical.

Frame 1195. Study the problem and solution in this frame.

DATA: Rx +1.50 +2.00 × 180 2^{Δ}B.U.

P.D. = 64
'A' Box = 48
'B' Box = 38
Dbl = 18

The horizontal decentration is 1 mm. **(in/out)**. The vertical decentration becomes:

$$V_d = \frac{10 \times \Delta}{P} = \frac{10 \times 2}{+3.50^*} = 5.7 \text{ mm. up}$$

**Note:* Power in vertical meridian.

The Optician decenters this lens 1 mm. in and 5.7 mm. **(up/down)**.

Answer 781. Made.

Frame 782. Visualize the Rx −4.00 +1.00 × 180 on the mental optical graph, as shown in this frame. This Rx is written in **(plus/minus)** cylinder.

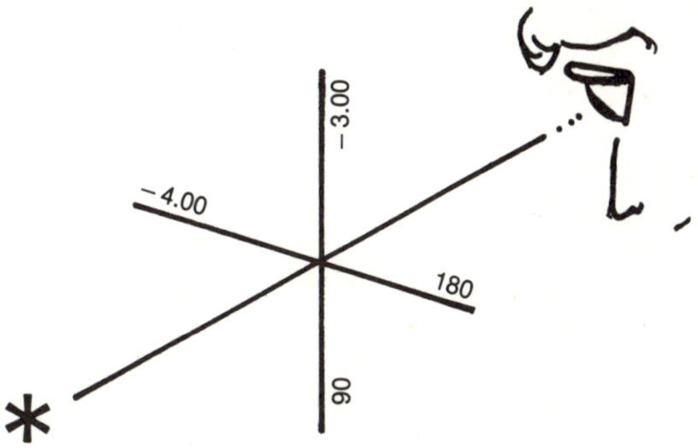

Answer 919. Two.

Frame 920. The amount of decentration multiplied by the lens power will equal the magnitude of created prism.

If the amount of decentration was 0.5 cm. and the power of the lens was +2.00 then 0.5 × 2.00 = 1.00Δ and the amount of prism is said to be 1.00 diopter.

This rule for the calculation of prism is a famous one in Opticianry. It was created by a man named Prentice.

That is why Opticians call it **(Prentice's/apprentices)** rule.

Answer 1057. B.D., two, non-similar or dissimilar.

Frame 1058. The third way an anisometropic Rx can be compensated is with the use of compensated segments. Consider the anatomy of a seg in this frame.

As you can see, by grinding the seg top or bottom away, the laboratory Optician **(can/cannot)** control the placement of the seg center.

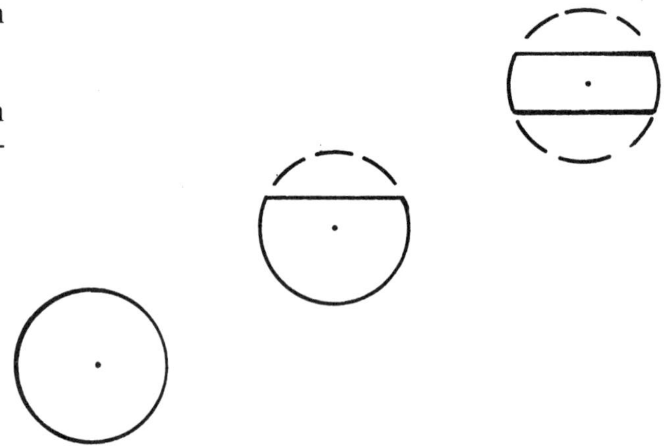

Answer 1195. In, up.

Frame 1196. Because prism Rx's are sometimes compounded, the Optician can solve by calculating each component separately to determine required decentration. Study the problem and solution in this frame.

Rx O.D. +2.00 +1.00 × 45 Δ 2 B.O. ⊙ 2 B.U.

P.D. = 64
'A' Box = 44
'B' Box = 34
Dbl = 20

P.D. Horizontal component:

$$\frac{(44+20)-(64)}{2}=0$$

Δ Horizontal component:

$$d=\frac{10\times\Delta}{P}=\frac{10\times 2}{+2.50}=8\text{ mm. out}$$

Δ Vertical component:

$$d=\frac{10\times\Delta}{P}=\frac{10\times 2}{+2.50}=8\text{ mm. up}$$

The layout is 8 mm. out and 8 mm. up **(O.D./O.S.)**.

Answer 782. Plus.

Frame 783. Even though the Rx is written in plus cylinder, the Optician may make (grind) the lens in **(plus/minus/both)** forms.

Plus form means the cylinder is on the front surface of the lens and minus cylinder means the cylinder is made on the **(back/edge)** of the lens.

Answer 920. Prentice's rule.

Frame 921. Prentice's rule states that prism (△) = decentration (d) in centimeters, times power (P). However, Opticians deal in **(meters/millimeters/centimeters)** and, therefore, require a modification of the Prentice rule.

Answer 1058. Can.

Frame 1059. The segment center can be controlled through manipulation of the top and bottom grinding. Study the examples in this frame.

The illustrations show seven different seg center placements through grinding. Which looks most like a base-up prism? **(4/9)**

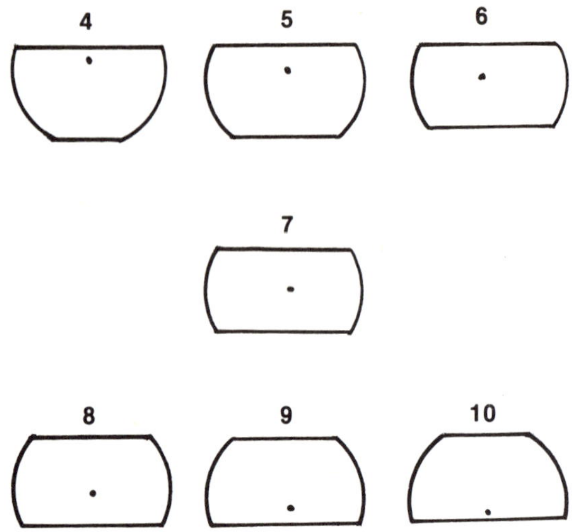

Answer 1196. O.D. (You gotta read carefully.)

Frame 1197. See if you can demonstrate your understanding of this Chapter by solving the compound problem in this frame. Compare your answers with the correct solutions in Frames 1198 and 1199.

DATA Rx O.D. −4.00 +2.00 × 135 2ΔB. I.
O.S. −5.00 +2.00 × 90 3ΔB.U.

P.D. = 65
'A' Box = 50
'B' Box = 40
Dbl = 20
E.D. = 54
O.C. = 3 Above or 23 High
Pattern
Measures = 51.5

Questions: What is the . . .

1. total decentration horizontal?
2. total decentration vertical?
3. Edger setting?

Answer 783. Both, Back.

Frame 784. The Rx −4.00 +1.00 × 180 may be ground in either plus or minus cylinder.

Study the illustrations in this frame. The illustrations show **(the same/different)** Rx's.

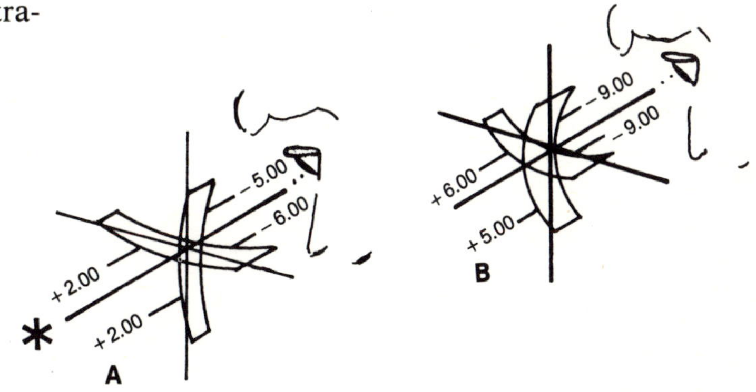

Answer 921. Millimeters.

Frame 922. Opticians use millimeters and, therefore, require modification of Prentice's rule.

Which example best represents the modification of Prentice's rule? **(A/B)**

A) $\Delta = d \times P$

B) $\Delta = \frac{d \times P}{10}$

Answer 1059. 4.

Frame 1060. The segment which most resembles a base-down prism is **(6/10)**.

Because these segments are ribbon-like in appearance, Opticians call them **(gibbon/ribbon)** segs.

Answer 1197. See answers below line.

Frame 1198. O.D.

1) What is total horizontal decentration?
   A. Decentration for P.D.
   B. Decentration for Δ.

A. $\frac{(50+20)-(65)}{2} = 2.5$ mm. in

B. $d = \frac{10 \times \Delta}{P} = \frac{10 \times 2}{-3.00} = 6.6$ mm. out

2.5 in + 6.6 out = 4.1 out

2) What is total vertical decentration?
   A. Decentration for O.C. Height
   B. Decentration for Δ.

A. $\frac{\text{'B' Box}}{2} - \text{O.C.} = \text{Vertical decentration}$

$\frac{40}{2} - 23 = 3$ mm. up

B. $d = \frac{10 \times \Delta}{P} = \frac{10 \times 0}{-3.00} = 0$ mm. up

3 mm. up + 0 mm. up = 3 mm. up

3) What should the Edger Set be?

$E_s = F_s - (P_s - 36.5)$
$E_s = 50 - (51.5 - 36.5)$
$E_s = 50 - 15$
$E_s = 36$

This Rx **(calls for/does not call for)** vertical prism.

Answer 784. Same.

Frame 785. The illustrations in Frame 784 show how −4.00 +1.00 × 180 is ground using plus cylinder form, and −3.00 −1.00 × 090 is ground using a minus cylinder form.

The total lens power illustrated in both A and B is **(the same/different).**

Answer 922. B. $\frac{d \times P}{10}$

Frame 923. By dividing the formula by 10, the conversion from centimeters to millimeters takes place. Test your knowledge of prism calculation by completing the chart below:

	decentration in mm.	×	Power	÷ 10	= Δ
Example:	3.0		3.00		.9
A)	5.0		5.00		?
B)	2.5		3.50		?
C)	6.0		6.75		?
D)	10.0		10.00		?

Answer 1060. 10, ribbon.

Frame 1061. Ribbon segs are available in seven styles with optical centers ranging from 4 Below seg top to 10 Below seg top. Their use is for imbalances less than 1.5 Δ and, therefore, is somewhat limited.

Because ribbon segs usually only compensate for 1.5 Δ or less, their use **(is/is not)** limited.

Answer 1198. Does Continue in next frame.

Frame 1199. O.S.

1) What is total horizontal decentration?
   A. Decentration for P.D.
   B. Decentration for Δ.

   A. $\frac{(50+20) - (65)}{2} = 2.5$ mm. in

   B. $d = \frac{10 \times \Delta}{P} = \frac{10 \times 0}{-3.00} = 0$ (none required)

   Total horizontal decentration = 2.5 mm. in

2) What is total vertical decentration?
   A. Decentration for O.C. or seg ht.
   B. Decentration for Δ.

   A. $\frac{\text{'B' Box}}{2} - \text{O.C.} = \text{Vertical decentration}$

   $\frac{40}{2} - 23 = 3$ mm. up

   B. $d = \frac{10 \times \Delta}{P} = \frac{10 \times 3}{-5.00} = \frac{30}{-5.00}$ 6 mm. down

   3 mm. up + 6 mm. down = 3 mm. down

3) What is Edger set?
   $E_s = F_s - (P_s - 36.5)$
   $E_s = 50 - (51.5 - 36.5)$
   $E_s = 50 - 15$
   $E_s = 36$

Does this Rx require oversize blanks? **(yes/no).**

Answer 785. The same.

Frame 786. $-4.00 + 1.00 \times 180$ is the same Rx as $-3.00 - 1.00 \times 090$. Study the illustration in this frame. The illustration shows a Rx already graphed on an optical cross on a visual line of sight.

Example **(A/B)** represents the same lens as seen through a lensometer.

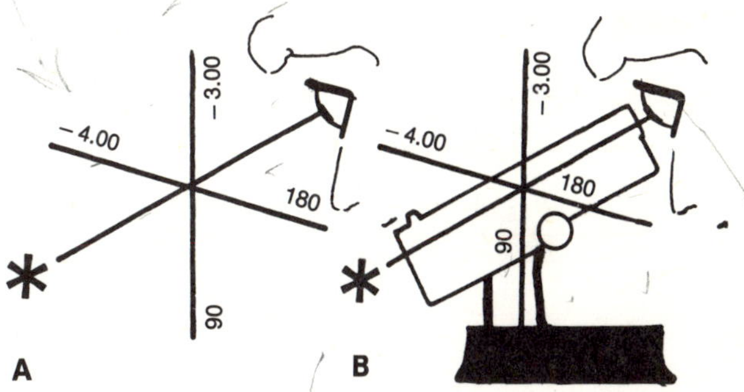

Answer 923. A) 2.5 Δ B) .875 Δ C) 4.05 Δ D) 10.0 Δ

Frame 924. The formula $\Delta = \frac{d \times P}{10}$ provides the Optician with the amount of prism as a result of decentration. Read the short optical story below.

The lab forgot to decenter the lenses for P.D. and the Optician looked at the data:

'A' Box	= 53
Dbl	= 18
P.D.	= 57
Rx	= −3.00

Failure to decenter creates a prismatic effect equal to the decentration that should have been performed. The needed decentration is **(7/9)** and the created prism, therefore, is **(2.1 Δ/2.7 Δ)**.

Answer 1061. Is.

Frame 1062. Study the Rx in this frame:

O.D. +2.00 +3.00 × 90
O.S. +2.00 +2.00 × 180 ADD +2.50
Reading Level 8 Below

$$\text{O.D.} = \Delta = \frac{d \times P}{10} = \frac{(8) \times (+2.00)}{10} = 1.6 \text{ B.U.}$$

$$\text{O.S.} = \Delta = \frac{d \times P}{10} = \frac{(8) \times (+4.00)}{10} = 3.2 \text{ B.U.}$$

To choose the correcting ribbon seg, the Optician must now determine what decentration (using the seg power) is needed to balance the prism:

$$\text{O.D. } d = \frac{10\,\Delta}{P} = \frac{(10) \times (1.6)}{+2.50} = 6.4 \text{ mm.}$$

$$\text{O.S. } d = \frac{10\,\Delta}{P} = \frac{(10) \times (3.2)}{+2.50} = 12.8 \text{ mm.}$$

The separation between the O.D. and O.S. seg center, then, must be 12.8 − 6.4 = 6.4 mm.

Answer 1199. No.

Frame 1200.

CHAPTER 19
TILT COMPENSATION

TURN TO THE BOTTOM OF PAGE 62, **FRAME 1201.**

Answer 786. B.

Frame 787. Example B in Frame 786 represents the lens as it would be positioned in a lensometer for neutralization. If the axis wheel was turned to 090°, the sphere meridian would read −3.00, and if the axis wheel was rotated to 180°, the sphere meridian would read **(−4.00/−1.00)**.

Answer 924. 7, 2.1 △.

Frame 925. Failure to decenter a −3.00 by 7 mm. created a prismatic effect of 2.1 △.

When decentration and lens power is known prism calculation is **(easy/hard)**.

Answer 1062. None required.

Frame 1063. The required seg separation is 6.4 mm. Look back at the choices of seg styles in Frame 1059. The two seg styles which have a 6 mm. separation (the closest to 6.4) are 4 and 10.

Which do you think is the correct solution, using compensated segs for the problem we have been working on? **(A/B)**

A) O.D. +2.00 +3.00 × 90
Compensated ribbon seg #4
O.S. +2.00 +2.00 × 180
Compensated ribbon seg #10
ADD +2.50

B) O.D. +2.00 +3.00 × 90
Compensated ribbon seg #3
O.S. +2.00 +2.00 × 180
Compensated ribbon seg #9
ADD +2.50

Answer 1200. None required.

Frame 1201. Opticians call frame tilt toward the cheeks *pantoscopic* and frame tilt away from the cheeks *retroscopic*. Study the examples in this frame.

Example **(A/B)** illustrates pantoscopic tilt.

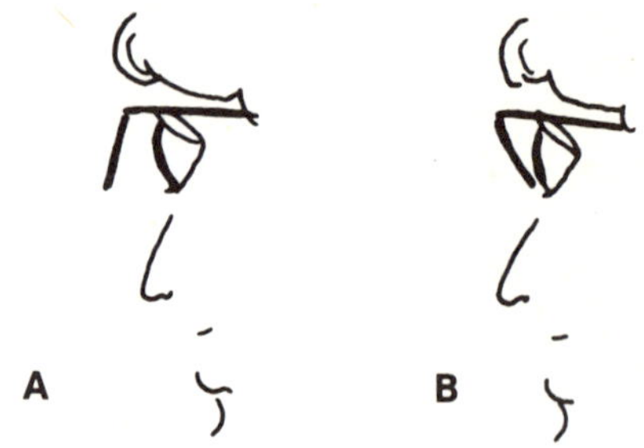

Answer 787. −4.00.

Frame 788. If the Optician was 'reading' the lens in Frame 786 and the first meridian of power found was −3.00, then the Optician would know this represented the sphere reading and record −3.00 ? × 090.

The next meridian to focus would be −4.00, representing the cylinder, and since the direction was minus, the cylinder would carry a minus sign and be correctly recorded as:
(−3.00 − 1.00 × 090/−3.00 + 4.00 × 090).

Answer 925. Easy. (If you said 'hard', read Volume I.)

Frame 926. When decentration and lens power are known, then prism calculation is easy. The consequence of decentration, that is, the prismatic effect, is then found.

Sometimes it may also be necessary for the Optician to calculate the amount of decentration necessary to create a needed amount of prism. Study the Rx in this frame.

The Rx **(calls for/does not call for)** prism.

Rx: +2.00 sph 5 △ Base In

Answer 1063. A. (There is no #3!)

Frame 1064. Review three out of the five ways you have learned to handle anisometropia in this Chapter.

1) Choose separate pairs of glasses: **(Reading+Sun/ Distance+Reading)**

2) Choose different seg styles or: **(similar/dissimilar)** segs.

3) Choose ribbon segs with **(the same/different)** seg O.C. heights.

Answer 1201. B.

Frame 1202. The effect of tilt on a prescription is minimal with respect to lower power or weak lenses.

Strong power lenses, however, **(can/cannot)** be effected.

Answer 788. **-3.00 -1.00×090.**

Frame 789. If, in Frame 786, the first meridian to focus was -4.00, the axis wheel would read 180 and the Rx would be read as -4.00 ? $\times$ 180. The next meridian found by turning the power wheel 'only' would read -3.00, so the Optician would know that the direction travelled on a number line was toward the **(minus/plus)** and the amount of travel was 1.00, therefore, resulting in a **(+1.00/ −1.00)**.

Would you record this as -4.00 $+1.00 \times$ **(180/090)**?

Answer 926. **Calls for.**

Frame 927. The Rx +2.00 sph 5 Δ B.I. calls for 5 diopters of prism. Can the Optician achieve this without special laboratory processing?

Study the prism formula once again. The formula must be solved for the (d) in the decentration formula. Which do you think is the correct formula to use? **(A/B)**

A) $\Delta = \dfrac{d \times P}{10}$ B) $d = \dfrac{10 \times \Delta}{P}$

Answer 1064. Reading+Distance, Dissimilar, Different.

Frame 1065. The fourth choice for aniso-metric management is the use of segments which already have prism in them. Opticians call these *Prism Segs*. Using Prism Segs for correction of vertical imbalances means either the tops or the bottoms of the segs will have thicker bases. Study the diagram in this frame.

From visual observation alone, which pair has Prism Segs? **(A/B)**

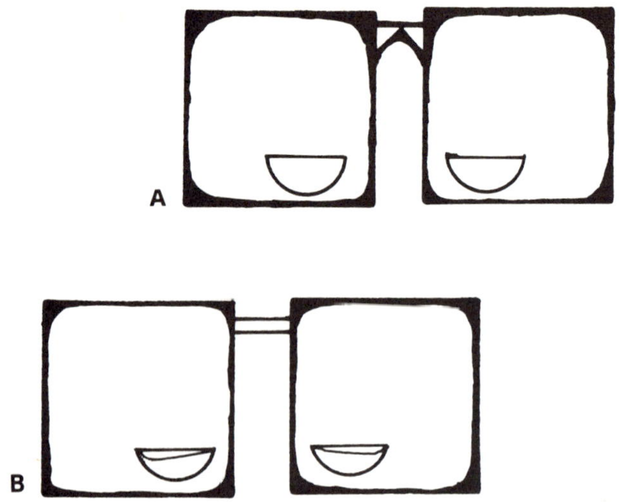

Answer 1202. Can.

Frame 1203. Strong power lenses are effected by tilt. Study the examples in this frame.

The lens most likely to be effected by tilt is **(A/B).**

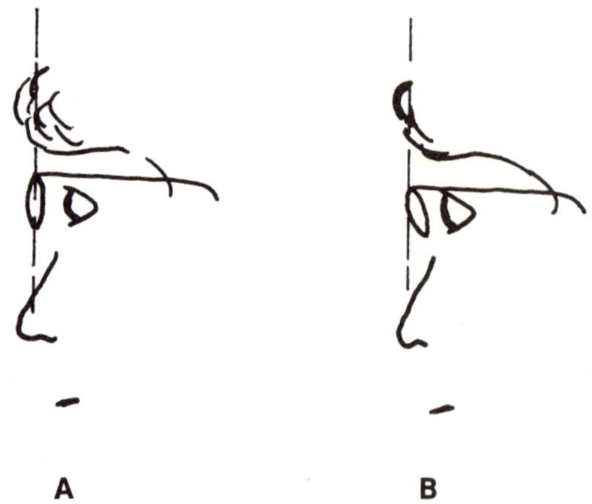

Answer 789. **Plus, +1.00, 180 *If you had difficulty with the last few frames, you may need to review Vol. I.**

Frame 790. Lens design continues with prescription analysis. By mentally visualizing a lens graphed on a visual line of sight or as if positioned in a lensometer, the Optician may understand how the power is distributed throughout the lens.

Lens design begins with a **(mental/dental)** visualization.

Answer 927. **B.**

Frame 928. The formula ten times the prism divided by the lens power equals the needed decentration. The Rx +2.00 sphere 5 Δ B.I. can now be "plugged in" to the formula $d = \frac{10 \times \Delta}{P}$ as follows:

d = decentration = ?
Δ = prism = 5.0
P = lens power = +2.00

$$d = \frac{10 \times 5.0}{2.00} = \frac{50.00}{2.00} = 25 \text{ mm.}$$

If the answer 25 mm. is correct, then it should fit the formula $\Delta = \frac{d \times P}{10}$ as proof. TRY IT!

Does $5.00\ \Delta = \frac{25 \times 2.00}{10}$? **(Yes/No)**

Answer 1065. B.

Frame 1066. Prism Segs are significantly thick and, therefore, cosmetically unappealing. The main advantage to Prism Segs is that they will compensate, for larger imbalances. Study the Rx in this frame:

O.D. −8.00
O.S. −2.00 ADD +2.50
Reading Level 7 Below

The prism imbalance is 4.2 Δ B.D. **(O.D./O.S.)**.

Answer 1203. B.

Frame 1204. Pantoscopic tilt affects both the sphere and the cylinder of strong prescriptions. In fact, tilt can induce (create) a cylinder where only a sphere Rx existed!

For example, 10° of Pantoscopic tilt on Rx +10.00 will result in the Rx +10.10 +0.31 × 180, to be exact. 20° of Pantoscopic tilt on a +10.00 sph will result in Rx +10.41 +1.38 × 180 to be exact.

Because Pantoscopic tilt is an integral part of ophthalmic dispensing, the Optician should learn to **(compensate/forget it)**.

Answer 790. Mental.

Frame 791. After mental visualization, the Optician adopts a criteria for how the lens is to be made.

This criteria begins with the lens form, that is, whether the lens is to be in plus or minus cylinder form.*

After mental visualization, the Optician adopts a **(criteria/cafeteria)** for how the lens is to be made.

*There is another form; crossed cylinder form that will be discussed later.

Answer 928. Yes. (Whew!)

Frame 929. Now consider an entire problem. Here is the data:

Eye Size 'A' Box = 52
Dbl = 18
P.D. = 61
E.D. = 55
Rx = +3.00 sph 3 △ B.I.

Question: 1) What is needed decentration for P.D.?
2) What is needed decentration for △ ?

Answer: 1) $\frac{(52+18) - (61)}{2} = 4.5$ mm.

2) $\frac{(10) \times (+3.00)}{+3.00} = 10$ mm.

The total needed decentration is the sum of steps one and two OR **(14.5/6.5)** millimeters.

Answer 1066. O.D.

Frame 1067. The correct Prism is one which can best cosmetically balance each side. Which do you think will *look* the best?

A) O.D. 3 B.U.
O.S. 1 B.D.

B) O.D. 4 B.U.
O.S. 0 B.D.

C) O.D. 2 B.U.
O.S. 2 B.D.

Answer 1204. Compensate.

Frame 1205. The formulation and calculation of the effect of any degree of pantoscopic tilt on a given Rx involves higher mathematics. The Optician, however, may use a general rule which helps to compensate for unwanted induced power of a strong Rx. The formula states: *lower the optical center 0.5 mm. for every 1° of pantoscopic tilt.*

For every one degree of pantoscopic tilt, the Optician should **(raise/lower)** the optical center one-half millimeter.

Answer 791. Criteria.

Frame 792. The criteria for lens design is: a lens that is optically (or) prescriptively correct, lightweight, thin as practical, and comfortable to the patient in its position in front of the eye.

Which is not a criteria for lens design?

1. Correct Rx
2. Lightweight
3. Thin as practical
4. Opticians name
5. Comfortable

Answer 929. 14.5

Frame 930. The total needed decentration for the problem in Frame 929 is 14.5 mm. Look at the data once again. Adding the E.D. to the total decentration means a minimum needed lens blank size of 55 + 14.5 or 69.5 mm.

If the Optician has a 70 mm. blank then this Rx **(may/may not)** be filled without special lab processing

Answer 1067. C

Frame 1068. The correct choice in balancing Vertical prism is a combination of Δ B.U. and Δ B.D. with as equal power possible. Prismatic Seg compensation, then, for the Rx is

O.D. −8.00 sph 2.0 B.U.
O.S. −2.00 sph 2.0 B.D.
ADD +2.50

Turn now to Frame 1069 for the fifth and final anisometropic tool for the Optician.

Answer 1205. Lower

Frame 1206. Because Opticians deal mostly in whole millimeters, the pantoscopic angle compensation formula can be practically modified. Which do you think expresses the formula correctly **(A/B)**?

A) Lower the O.C. 1 mm. for every 2° of angle.
B) Lower the O.C. 2 mm. for every 1° of angle.

Answer 792. **4.**

Frame 793. Lens design begins with base curve selection. Whereas, there are many formulas for lens curvature, Opticians know that patients can become accustomed to certain base curves. We are all creatures of habit, therefore:

Being accustomed to a certain base curve can become a **(habit/habbit)**, and changing the base curve may cause **(necessary/unnecessary)** adaptive changes on the part of the patient.

Answer 930. **may**

Frame 931. Special lab processing may mean the incorporation of prism into the Rx itself or it may mean the use of extra large lens blanks. Opticians call extra large lens blanks "oversize blanks" and the incorporation of prism "prism grinding".

Do you think it is possible for a given Rx to need both prism grinding and oversize blanks? **(yes/no)**

Answer 1068. None required . . . please continue.

Frame 1069. You have seen, thus far, that this business of compensation for anisometropias in multifocals is one of optical center management (no pun intended). Thus far, you have worked with existing forms, that is, single vision, flat top, round top, ultex and executive, ribbon, and prism segs; all of which had fixed optical centers.

The fifth form for the Optician is one in which another O.C. is created thus yielding a lens with not one, but **(three/two)** centers.

Answer 1206. A

Frame 1207. The Optician should lower the O.C. 1 mm. for every 2° of pantoscopic angle.

Study the problem in this frame. O.C. should be lowered 3.5 mm. This is best illustrated as **(A/B)**.

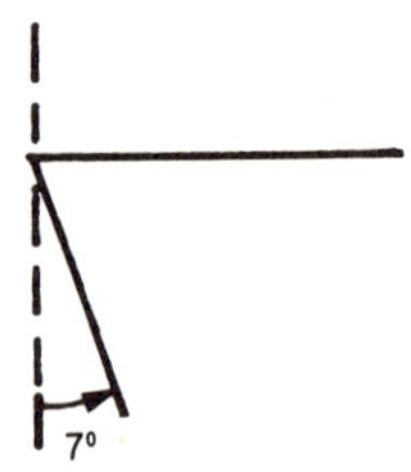

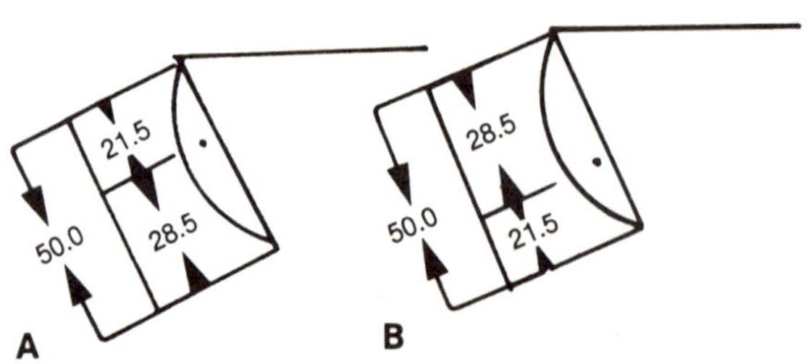

Answer 793. Habit, unnecessary

. . . .

Frame 794. Patients often develop a habit of becoming accustomed to a certain base curve. Changing the base curve may often force a **(change/chain)** in habit.

The selection of the correct base curve is dependent upon two major factors.

Base curve selection is dependent upon **(one/two)** major factors.

Answer 931. yes

. . . .

Frame 932. The Optician can judge whether prism grinding or oversize blanks is necessary by understanding the prism and decentration formulas. You have noticed that so far all the problems in this Chapter on decentration and prism have been simple prescriptions; that is, spheres only.

With compound lenses, another element is added. Compound Rx's are **(the same/different)** than sphere Rx's.

Answer 1069. Two

Frame 1070. In optics, the word for two is bi. Therefore, the grinding of two different optical centers may be called **(bicentric/monocentric)** grinding.

Answer 1207. B

Frame 1208. The pantoscopic angle compensation formula applies to stronger prescriptions. (approximately 7.00 diopters and higher.) However, patients may complain of asthenopia (discomfort) with prescriptions lower than 7.00 diopters which can be helped with tilt and compensation.

As a rule, whenever the Rx is greater than plus or minus five diopters, the Optician should think about tilt effect and the pantoscopic compensation formula with reference to the frame angle and the **(seg. ht/OC)**.

Answer 794. Change, Two

Frame 795. The two major factors of base curve selection are:

The previous (or previously comfortable) base curve, and the power of the new lens.

The power of the lens may dictate the base curve because the new curvature may be impossible with the old base curve. If the new Rx was −3.00 +5.50 × 180 and the old Rx was on a plus two base, the new Rx in minus cylinder form would be **(possible/impossible)** on a +2.00 Base.

Answer 932. different

Frame 933. Compound Rx's differ from sphere Rx's when it comes to the prism and decentration formulas. Study the Rx in this frame:

−2.00 +3.00 × 180

P D = 65
'A' Box = 55
Dbl = 18
E D = 58

Question: What is the consequence of failure to decenter for P.D.?

Answer: Since P.D. decentration is **(horizontal/vertical)**, the Optician must first calculate the power in that meridian.

Answer 1070. Bicentric

. . . .

Frame 1071. Opticians call bicentric grinding by its optical nickname: Slab Off. Slab Off gets its name from a step in its fabrication, namely, a thin slice or slab of material which is ground off.

Study the example in this frame. The illustration shows the fabrication of a Slab **(Off/On).**

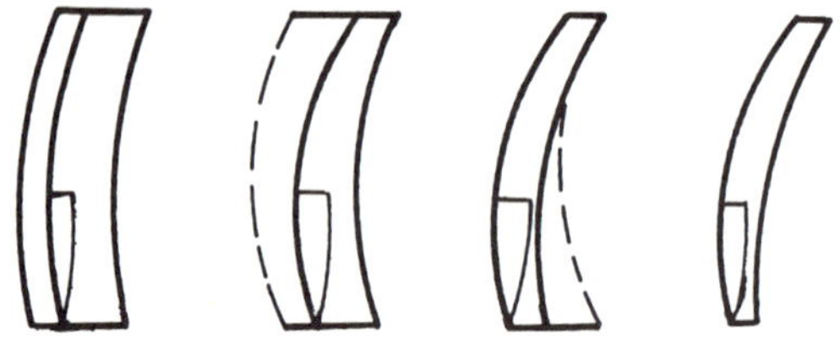

Answer 1208. O.C.

. . . .

Frame 1209.

CHAPTER 20
COLOR AND LIGHT

TURN TO THE BOTTOM OF PAGE 80, **FRAME 1210.**

Answer 795. Impossible (in minus cylinder form)

Frame 796. The Rx −3.00 +5.50 × 180 is not possible in conventional minus cylinder form using a +2.00 Base. Study the illustration in this frame.

The needed back curve in the vertical meridian would have to be **(plus/minus).**

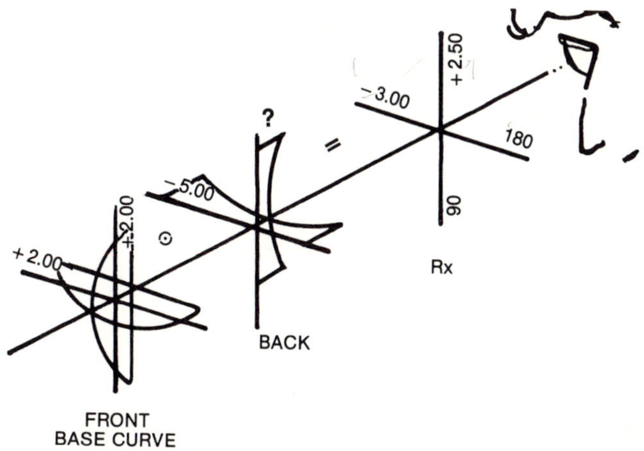

Answer 933. horizontal (If you had difficulty with that answer, please re-read Chapter 2).

Frame 934. When considering horizontal decentration for P.D., the Optician must use the power in the horizontal meridian. Look at the Rx once again: −2.00 +3.00 × 180

Power in the horizontal meridian is (−2.00/+3.00).

Answer 1071. Off.

Frame 1072. Slab Off is always ground base up in glass, but can be ground base up **or** base down in plastic. Study the Rx and data in this frame:

O.D. +2.00 +2.00 × 180
O.S. +1.50 +1.00 × 180 ADD +2.50
Reading level 10 mm. below, glass flat top bifocals.

$$\text{O.D. } \Delta = \frac{d \times P}{10} = \frac{(10) \times (+4.00)}{10} = 4.0 \text{ B.U.}$$

$$\text{O.S. } \Delta = \frac{d \times P}{10} = \frac{(10) \times (+2.50)}{10} = 2.5 \text{ B.U.}$$

TOTAL VERTICAL Δ = 1.5 B.U. O.D.

The Slab Off to be ordered will be base up and ordered on the lens to most balance the prism. Since adding more B.U. to the O.D. would worsen the situation, the obvious answer is slab off the **(O.D./O.S.)**

Answer 1209. None required.

Frame 1210. Even though lenses are transparent, they absorb and reflect some light. Study the diagrams in this frame.

The diagrams illustrate **(3/5)** different ways light can reflect as it passes through a lens.

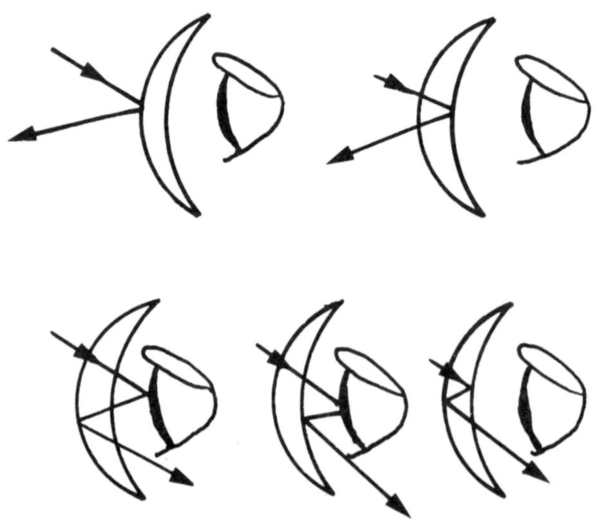

Answer 796. Plus.

Frame 797. The concave vertical meridian of a −3.00 +5.50 × 180 on a +2.00 Base would have to be plus, which is impossible in meniscus form.

The logical base curve for this prescription then, would be one in which the concave vertical meridian could be **(minus/plus/plano).** That base curve could be **(+2.50/+3.00)** base.

Answer 934. −2.00.

Frame 935. In order to avoid confusion, the formulas for prism and decentration should be further clarified. Study the modified prism and decentration formulas in the frame.

$$\Delta = \frac{d \times P_{\text{(in the meridian in question)}}}{10}$$

AND

$$d = \frac{10\,\Delta}{P_{\text{(in the meridian in question)}}}$$

The meridian in question in Frame 933 is horizontal so the correct power to be used as P is **(−2.00/+1.00).**

Answer 1072. O.S.

Frame 1073. Because slab off creates a base up prism in the seg only, without disturbing the distance, it is ground on the lens that has the weakest plus or strongest minus in the vertical meridian. Study the example in the frame:

Rx O.D. −1.00 −1.00 × 180
O.S. −5.00 −1.00 × 180 ADD +2.50
Reading level 8 mm below

The lens with the weakest plus or strongest minus is **(O.D./O.S.)** and should have a slab off of 3.0 Δ **(B.U./B.D.)**

Answer 1210. 5

Frame 1211. Because reflections can come from both front and back surfaces of a lens, the Optician, who treats only one side may still encounter problems with the **(edge/other side).**

Answer 797. Minus, +3.00

Frame 798. An Optician could spend many hours computing and calculating lens design based upon a given base curve. Fortunately, optical scientists have already established the most workable curves for any given prescription. These curves have been placed in chart form.

The optical scientist has saved the Optician from personally having to calculate **(base curves/bottled coors).**

Answer 935. −2.00

Frame 936. When calculating the consequence of failing to decenter the Rx −2.00 +3.00 × 180, when P D = 65, 'A' Box = 55, Dbl = 18, the correct formula to use is **(A/B)**.

A) $\Delta = \dfrac{4 \times -2.00}{10}$

B) $\Delta = \dfrac{4 \times +3.00}{10}$

Answer 1073. O.S., B.U.

Frame 1074. Because all five methods of solving vertical prismatic anisometropia requires alteration of the Doctor's prescription, the Optician should **(ignore/consult)** with the Doctor before proceeding.

Answer 1211. Other side.

Frame 1212. Because of reflections and absorbtion of some light, the 100% available light is reduced to approximately 92%. Opticians call the precent of light that travels completely through a lens its "transmission".

Do you think the transmission of clear ordinary crown glass is **(8%/92%)**?

Answer 798. Base curves.

Frame 799. If the patient has had no previous base curve, or the Rx is the patient's first, the Optician can choose a curve from charts. Base curve charts are usually available from the laboratory Optician, however, in their absence, the Optician may use a simple formula.

The Base Curve formula is presented in Chapter 6, Frame 854.

Please continue with the Lens Design on the next page, Frame 800.

Answer 936. A

Frame 937. Answer A is correct. Because the axis meridian is **(important/unimportant)**, the Optician must have the ability to calculate the power of any lens in a given meridian, especially the decentration meridians of 90 and 180. This subject continues in Chapter 11 — CYLINDER ANALYSIS.

Answer 1074. Consult.

Frame 1075. Test your knowledge of compensating for vertical imbalances at the reading level by choosing the correct answers.

Anisometropia in multifocals **(may/may not)** be compensated for in five ways. These imbalances occur as the visual line of sight tracks **(horizontally/vertically)** from primary gaze to some point in the seg. The Optician must first calculate the total lens power at **(180/90)** and then multiply, using the formula ($\Delta = \frac{d \times P}{10}$/$\Delta$ **d × P)** for each eye. The net effect of this prism is the amount of **(vertical/oblique)** prism. The first method eliminates the need for multifocals and is **(one good/two)** pairs of glasses.

Answer 1212. 92%.

Frame 1213. With the application of color or coating, this transmission can be either improved or reduced. By applying a special anti-reflective coating to the lens, for example, some of the reflections can be eliminated, thereby improving a clear lens from 92% transmission to as high as 98% transmission. Both glass and plastic lenses may be treated for enhancement or reduction of light transmission. Some lenses, such as photochromic, even have a built-in transmission control.

(All/Some) lenses have built-in transmission control.

Answer 799. **No answer required. Go to Frame 800.**

Frame 800. In the beginning of this section, the criteria for lens design was stated. This criteria consists of 1) The correct Rx. 2) As thin and lightweight a lens as practical, and 3) Comfortable to wear.

The Optician knows that the choice of lens material can affect the resultant lens. So the first consideration of lens materials is to be the index of refraction.

Index of refraction is the **(first/third)** consideration of lens material.

Answer 937. **important**

Frame 938.

CHAPTER 11
CYLINDER ANALYSIS

TURN TO THE BOTTOM OF PAGE 89, **FRAME 939**

Answer 1075. **May, Vertical, 90°, $\Delta = \frac{d \times P}{10}$, Vertical, Two.**

Frame 1076. A second method of using segments of different styles is called **(compensated prism/dissimilar)** segs. This second method can compensate for **(small/large)** imbalances. Thirdly, the Optician can select the use of **(ribbon/ribeye)** segs which have one of **(six/seven)** different optical centers. The fourth choice utilized segs **(without/with)** prism ground into them and where as these **(Prism/Prison)** Segs can compensate for **(large/medium)** imbalances, they are generally considered to be un-**(cosmetic/healthy)**. The fifth method available to the Optician involves creating **(one/two)** centers.

Answer 1213. **Some.**

Frame 1214. The application of color reduces the transmission of lenses. Although color can greatly reduce unwanted light (glare), it can also affect transmission enough to create an uncomfortable or even dangerous situation.

A person driving at night with sunglasses to reduce the bothersome glare from oncoming cars is **(lowering/raising)** the transmission to a **(safe/dangerous)** level.

Answer 800. **first**

Frame 801. Index of refraction is the first consideration of lens material. The Index of Refraction is an optical expression for a ratio. A ratio, by definition, is one thing compared to another. For example: flat tops to round tops.

A ratio is **(nothing/one thing)** compared to another.

Answer 938. **none required**

Frame 939. The Optician sometimes needs to be able to identify the power of a cylinder in a meridian other than its own axis in order to calculate prismatic effect. Study the Rx in this frame.

Rx: −2.50 +3.00 × 90

The Rx −2.50 +3.00 × 90 has **(−2.50/+3.00)** at 90 and **(+3.00/+0.50)** at 180.

Answer 1076. Dissimilar, Large, Ribbon, Seven, With, Prism, Large, Cosmetic, Two.

Frame 1077. Another method is creating an additional Optical Center **(with/without)** changing the distance Rx. Slab **(Off/On)** is ground only **(B.D./B.U.)** in glass, but may be ground **(B.D./B.U.)** in plastic. The Optician Slabs Off the **(stronger/weaker)** plus or the **(weaker/stronger)** minus. For the Rx:

O.D. +3.00 +2.00 × 45 ADD +3.00
O.S. +2.00 +1.50 × 90
READING LEVEL 8 BELOW

The total vertical imbalance is **(6.1/1.6)** **(B.D./B.U.)** in front of **(O.D./O.S.)** and **(may/may not)** be slabbed off with **(B.U./B.D.)** in the **(O.D./O.S.)**.

Answer 1214. Lowering, dangerous.

Frame 1215. Color, by itself, reduces transmission but may allow harmful light rays, such as ultraviolet, to pass through the lens. The Optician can choose the appropriate lens color by understanding not only its transmission of all light, but its transmission of selected types of light such as ultraviolet or infrared, as well.

All light is **(the same/different)**.

Answer 801. One thing.

Frame 802. A ratio is one thing compared to another. Study the example in this frame. The example illustrates 3 ratios.

Which ratio do you think applies to Opticianry? **(A/B/C).**

A. $\dfrac{\textbf{The thickness of one piece.}}{\textbf{The thickness of another piece.}}$

B. $\dfrac{\textbf{The weight of one apple.}}{\textbf{The weight of another apple.}}$

C. $\dfrac{\textbf{The speed of light in one substance.}}{\textbf{The speed of light in another substance.}}$

Answer 939. −2.50 × 90 +0.50 × 180.

Frame 940. Because the Rx −2.50 +3.00 × 90 is −2.50 at 90 and +0.50 at 180, the Optician would use **(+0.50/ −2.50)** to represent P in the horizontal decentration formula. Choose the correct statement in this frame.

If the P.D. is off by 6 mm, then the Optician calculates the prismatic result by using the formula **(A/B).**

A) $\Delta = \dfrac{-2.50 \times 6}{10}$

B) $\Delta = \dfrac{+0.50 \times 6}{10}$

Answer 1077. Without, off, up, B.D., weaker, stronger, 1.6, B.U., O.D., may, B.U., O.S.

Frame 1078. When anisometropic imbalances are calculated for compound lenses with oblique axis, the Optician must use the same guidelines as in Frames 997, 998, Chapter 12. Study the example in this frame. The example illustrates an Rx with **(oblong/oblique)** axis.

O.D. +0.50 +1.00 × 135 ADD +2.25
O.S. +3.00 +2.50 × 30
Reading level 8 mm. below

Without trigonometry, the calculation which would compute the precise (vertical and horizontal) compounded effects of induced prism at oblique axis, the answers arrived at by multiplying the difference between the vertical O.D. [+0.50 + (50% of +1.00) = +1.00] and the vertical O.S. [+3.00 + (75% of +2.50) = 4.87] or (+4.87) − (+1.00) = 3.87.

$$3.87 \times 8 = \frac{30.96}{10} = 3.09\ \Delta$$ B.U. O.S., would be **(absolutely accurate/close enough)**.

Answer 1215. Different.

Frame 1216. Through the study of transmission charts, the Optician can tell what type of light is transmitted at what level. Study the chart in this frame. The chart shows **(two/one)** wave length(s).

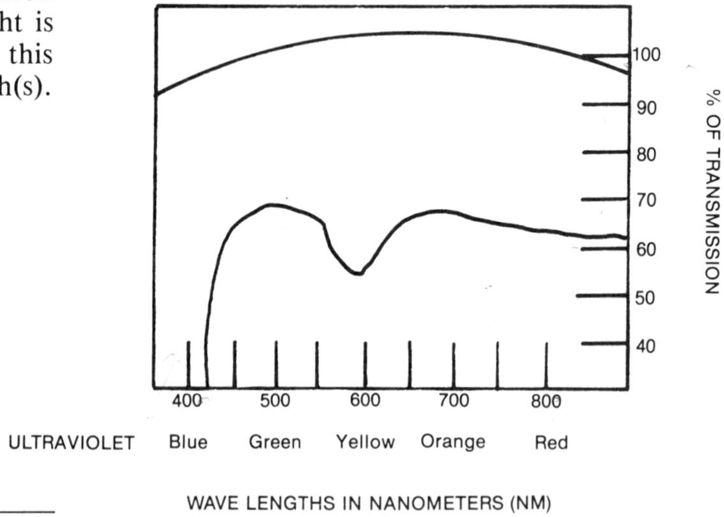

Answer 802. **C**

Frame 803. Example C:

$$\frac{\text{The speed of light in one substance.}}{\text{The speed of light in another substance.}}$$

is a ratio relative to optics.

This ratio is read: "The speed of light in one substance compared to the speed of light in another substance".

Opticians are interested in a special ratio known as the **(index of refraction/index of retraction).**

Answer 940. **+0.50, B (P.D. is horizontal)**

Frame 941. Now, consider the Rx +3.00 −1.00 × 180, 2 Δ B.U. This Rx calls for prism base up. So, the Optician must use the **(horizontal/vertical)** meridian for the decentration formula. Do you think the correct formula is represented by **(A/B/C)**?

A) $d = \frac{10 \times 2}{+3.00}$

B) $d = \frac{10 \times 2}{-1.00}$

C) $d = \frac{10 \times 2}{+2.00}$

Answer 1078. Oblique, close enough

Frame 1079. For purposes of deciding whether or not a given Rx with oblique axis has sufficient prismatic imbalance to require compensation, the Optician may use the formula $\Delta = \frac{d \times P}{10}$ in the given meridian. For purposes of exact mathematical answers, the Optician should learn **(Trigonometry/Astronomy).**

Answer 1216. Two

Frame 1217. By referring to transmission charts, the Optician can find the correct lens for a given situation. Dark lenses may reduce illumination but they do not always reduce transmission of such harmful rays as ultraviolet and infrared.

Colored lenses such as non-optical store bought sunglasses reduce illumination due to the density of the color, but offer **(good/little)** harmful ray protection.

Answer 803. Index of Refraction.

Frame 804. The index of refraction is found by the ratio of

$$\frac{\text{The speed of light in air.}}{\text{The speed of light in a particular lens material.}}$$

This is correctly read as, "the speed of light in air **(compared/rated)** to the speed of light in a particular lens material.

Answer 941. Vertical, C. If you missed this, please re-read Chapter 2 thru 4.

Frame 942. The power at 90, of the Rx +300 −1.00 × 180 is +2.00. Therefore, the answer C in Frame 941 is correct.

When the axis of the cylinder is 90 or 180, the power in each respective meridian is easily calculated. When the axis is oblique, that is, other than 90 or 180, the formula becomes more complex.

Oblique axes require **(more/less)** complex formulas.

Answer 1079. Trigonometry

Frame 1080.

CHAPTER 15
ANISEIKONIA AND MAGNIFICATION

TURN TO THE TOP OF PAGE 98, **FRAME 1081.**

Answer 1217. No

Frame 1218. Lens color can be applied over an existing clear lens or it may be placed within the lens at the time of manufacture. Some lenses have special filters placed in them during the manufacture cycle which acts as a super ultraviolet or infrared absorber.

When color or coating is applied to these lenses, protection is **(enhanced/diminished).**

Answer 804. compared

Frame 805. The expression

$$\frac{\text{speed of light in air}}{\text{speed of light in a particular material}}$$ is read

"The speed of light in air compared to the speed of light in a particular lens material."

The index of refraction is a mathematical formula. Study the examples in this frame. Example **(A/B)** represents the correct formula for index of refraction.

A. $\text{Index of Refraction} = \dfrac{\text{Speed of light in lens}}{\text{Speed of light in air}}$

B. $\text{Index of Refraction} = \dfrac{\text{Speed of light in air}}{\text{Speed of light in lens}}$

____

Answer 942. more (you wouldn't think it would get easier would you?)

Frame 943. The mathematical computations required to calculate the precise cylinder power at any point from its original axis requires the skill of geometry and trigonometry. This book uses a somewhat less precise, but still very useful method which foregoes the gymnastics of higher mathematics.

Geometry, Trigonometry and **(other/no other)** methods exist for oblique cylinder analysis.

____

Answer 1080. None required

Frame 1081. When significant differences between the prescriptions of two eyes are present, the difference in the image sizes seen by the brain can cause problems.

Significant differences in image sizes "seen" by the brain **(can/cannot)** cause problems.

Answer 1218. enhanced.

Frame 1219. Coating is usually applied under a vacuum where the lens is first placed in a chamber. The air is then withdrawn from the chamber to create a vacuum whereupon a capsule of color or coating material is released and under pressure adheres to the lens surface.

Another way to achieve color is the process of tinting a lens. Color can be achieved through coating and **(tainting/tinting).**

Answer 805. B

Frame 806. The formula for Index of Refraction is:

$$\text{Index of Refraction} = \frac{\text{Speed of light in air}}{\text{Speed of light in lens}}$$

Opticians use the symbol (n) for the index of refraction.

The symbol for index of refraction is **(n/N).**

Answer 943. other

Frame 944. The Optician can construct a chart, which if kept at the dispensing table, may be quickly referenced to solve oblique axis prescription problems.

Oblique axis prescription problems may be solved with the use of a **(chart/chard).**

Answer 1081. Can

Frame 1082. Opticians know that the eye acts like a camera; light rays focused upon the retina form an image, which in turn, is transmitted to the brain for interpretation. When the prescription between two eyes are significantly different that the image sizes seen by the brain are **(never/also)** different.

Answer 1219. Tinting

Frame 1220. Tinting is a dye and bleach process which can be performed upon plastic lenses only.* Plastic lenses are immersed into hot dye solutions which allow the dye to become absorbed. The greater the absorbtion, the darker the color.

Opticians who wish to control ultraviolet and/or infrared transmissions, must first understand the transmission effects of the dyes used.

If a moral for this Chapter had to be written, it could be "All that glitters is not **(sold/gold)**."

*At the time of the writing of this book.

Answer 806. **n**

Frame 807. The index of refraction symbol is a lower case N or n. The formula then is:

$$n = \frac{\text{Speed of light in air}}{\text{Speed of light in glass}}$$

The speed of light in air is learned by everyone at an early age. Do you remember if this is **(186,000 miles per second/186,000 miles per hour)?***

*Hint: Light travels very fast.

Answer 944. **chart**

Frame 945. The key to the oblique axis chart construction is the number

1 2 4 5 6 7 8 8 9 9 8 8 7 6 5 4 2 1 .

Step One is to memorize that number.

At first glance, this seems **(hard/easy)**.

Answer 1082. Also

Frame 1083. Study the Rx's in this frame:

A. O.D. +5.00 sph
O. S. +0.75 sph   Add +2.00

B. O.D. −5.00 sph
O. S. −0.75 sph   Add +2.00

Since plus magnifies and minus minifies, which do you suppose creates a larger retinal image, Rx **(A/B)**?

Answer 1220. Gold

Frame 1221.

CHAPTER 21
SAFETY LENSES

TURN TO PAGE 104, **FRAME 1222.**

Answer 807. 186,000 miles per second. Good for you!

Frame 808. In the formula for index of refraction, the speed of light in air is always the top number of the ratio or 186,000. The speed of light in regular glass happens to be 122,000 miles per second. Therefore, the formula to be solved becomes

$$\left(n = \frac{186{,}000}{122{,}000} \quad / \quad n = \frac{122{,}000}{186{,}000} \right)$$

Unless you enjoy long division, go get a calculator and then turn to Frame 809, on the top of Page 105. I'll wait.

Answer 945. hard (it really is easy!)

Frame 946. Look again at the key to oblique axis chart construction. The number 1 2 4 5 6 7 8 8 9 9 8 8 7 6 5 4 2 1 has two unique features about it.

This number has **(one/two)** unique features about it.

Answer 1083. A

Frame 1084. Rx A in Frame 1083 creates a larger retinal image. Rx B is minus and would therefore create a smaller image.

Look back at Frame 1083 once again. The lens which will create the smallest image is **(A, O.S./B, O.S.)** and the lens which will create the largest image is **(A, O.D./B, O.D.)**

Answer 1221. None Required.

Frame 1222. As Opticianry reaches the age of accountability, it also assumes responsibility for the products it dispenses. The safety and security of lenses and frames is one of those responsibilities.

Opticians are responsible to society for the products it **(disperses/dispenses).**

Answer 808. $n = \frac{186{,}000}{122{,}000}$ **You didn't have to rush.**

Frame 809. Solve the formula $n = \frac{186{,}000}{122{,}000}$ by dividing 186,000 by 122,000.

Your answers should read 1.52. This means that the index of refraction for regular glass is 1.52.

If the speed of light in other materials were known, the Optician **(could/could not)** find their index of refraction also.

Answer 946. **two**

Frame 947. The number 1 2 4 5 6 7 8 8 9 9 8 8 7 6 5 4 2 1 has two unique features about it. The first unique feature is that the number is a mirror of 1 2 4 5 6 7 8 8 9 where the other half of the mirror is **(9 8 8 7 6 5 4 2 1 / 1 2 3 4 5 6 7 8 9 10)**

Answer 1084. B O.S., A O.D.

Frame 1085. Image sizes which are unequal are called aniseikonic. The greek work "iso" means equal and the greek word "konia" means shape, and the "an" means not.

Therefore, aniseikonia must mean **(equal/unequal)** shapes.

Answer 1222. Dispenses

Frame 1223. Safety of eyewear subdivides into two categories: Industrial and Street Wear.

Laws governing industrial eyewear state that the lenses must be of sufficient strength to withstand the impact of a 1" steel ball dropped from a height of 50 inches, without the lens breaking. The laws for industrial safety also state that the minimum thickness of the lens be 3 mm.

For minus lenses, the center must be 3 mm. and for plus lenses, the **(center/edge)** must meet the 3 mm. standard. There are **(one/two)** requirements for industrial safety lenses.

Answer 809. could

Frame 810. Test your knowledge of how to find the index of refraction of the following materials from the information below.

A. $n = \dfrac{186{,}000}{110{,}000}$

B. $n = \dfrac{186{,}000}{122{,}000}$

The answers appear in the next frame.

Answer 947. 9 8 8 7 6 5 4 2 1

Frame 948. The "mirror" of 9 8 8 7 6 5 4 2 1 is 1 2 4 5 6 7 8 8 9. The number then to memorize becomes instantly easier because there are really only 9 numbers to remember instead of **(18/12).**

Answer 1085. Unequal

Frame 1086. Opticians know that aniseikonia deals with the image size differences, that is, the magnification or minification of images caused by plus and minus lenses.

When lens powers are very unequal, or aniseikonic, the Optician may balance one image size to another by increasing the magnification of one lens while reducing the magnification of the **(other/another).**

Answer 1223. Edge, Two

Frame 1224. Street wear safety requires only that a lens be able to withstand the impact of 5/8'' steel ball dropped from a height of 50 inches without the lens breaking.

Lenses which are exempt from the ''dropball'' rule, are those which have sharp edges, such as executive multifocals. Plastic lenses are also exempt because they are inherently impact resistant.

Study the illustration in this frame. Lens **(A/B)** is exempt from the dropball test.

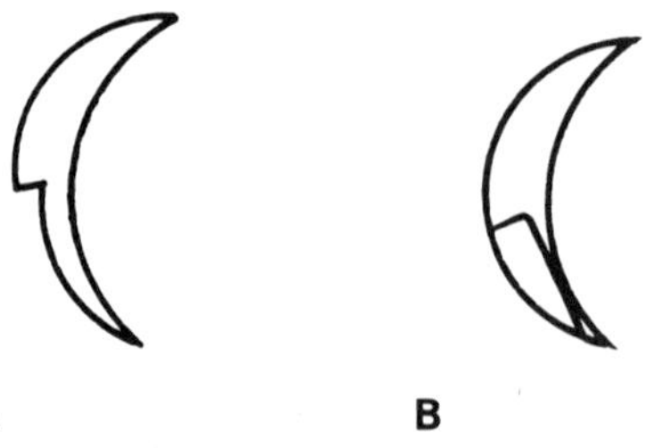

Answer 810. A. 1.69 B. 1.52

Frame 811. It is important to remember that in Optics, index and thickness are opposites. The higher the index, the **(thinner/thicker)** the lens.

In Optics, thickness and index are **(opposites/the same).**

Answer 948. 18

Frame 949. A nine number digit is as simple as your area code plus a telephone number. Complete the "mirror" of the number in this frame. The number is 1 2 4 5 6 7 8 8 9 ________________. and check your answer.

Answer 1086. Other

Frame 1087. Study the Rx in this frame.

O.D. +10.00 +1.00 × 180
O.S. + 6.00 +1.00 × 90

Because the magnification of the O.D. is greater, the Optician might wish to balance this Rx by **(increasing/decreasing)** the magnification of the O.D. and **(decreasing/increasing)** the magnification of the O.S.

Answer 1224. A

Frame 1225. Glass lenses may be rendered impact resistant by either one of two methods: Thermal (heat), or Chemical Strengthening. Thermal (heat) strengthening uses an oven to bring the lens close to its melting point. The lens is then ejected and rapidly cooled with air jets. Because the outside is being cooled at a different rate than the inside, stress is set up forming a case around the lens.

Since the case offers a hard protection for the lens, Opticians call this method **(case hardened/case protection)**

Answer 811. thinner, opposites

. . . .

Frame 812. "The higher the index number, the thinner the lens" is an optical rule. Look back at the answers to Frame 810

The two numbers were **(1.52, 1.69/1.94, 9.16)**

____

Answer 949. 1 2 4 5 6 7 8 8 9 - 9 8 8 7 6 5 4 2 1.

. . . .

Frame 950. Your answer should match 1 2 4 5 6 7 8 8 9 - 9 8 8 7 6 5 4 2 1. Just for the fun of it, close your eyes and try to repeat from memory, the sequence of numbers just illustrated. You'll be surprised at how well you will do.

____

Answer 1087. decreasing, increasing

Frame 1088. This business of magnification in lenses depends upon two different factors. Factor number one is the magnification caused by the lens curvature (base curve), and factor number two, is the lens thickness at its center.

Since these two properties affect the shape of a lens, the magnification factor is called **(shape/shade)** magnification factor.

Answer 1225. Case hardened

Frame 1226. Chemical strengthening renders a lens impact resistant by immersing it in a chemical bath for a prolonged period (usually 15 hours) which causes a salt ion exchange to occur. The completion of this chemical exchange is what renders the lens impact resistant.

The time difference between the thermal and chemical process is significant. Which do you think takes longer, **(chemical/thermal)**?

Answer 812. 1.52, 1.69

Frame 813. The index of refraction of regular glass is 1.52. The index of refraction of plastic is 1.49, and the index of refraction of hilite or high index glass is 1.69.

Using your knowledge of the "index rule of opposites", which lens will be thinner **(1.49** or **1.52)**?

____

Answer 950. 1 2 4 5 6 7 8 8 9 - 9 8 8 7 6 5 4 2 1.

Frame 951. Back in Frame 946, you were told that there were two unique features about the number 1 2 4 5 6 7 8 8 9 9 8 8 7 6 5 4 2 1 . One feature was the mirror image of the easily memorized nine digit number, and the second unique feature is the absence of a sequential number.

Look again at the number. **HINT. The missing digit in the beginning sequence rhymes with tree. The number is **(three/ten)**.

____

Answer 1088. shape factor

Frame 1089. The shape factor is the result of both the base curve and the lens thickness. The second factor for magnification is the effect of the lens power, plus the distance this power sits from the eye (vertex distance).

Because this concerns power, Opticians call this second factor the **(Power/Powder)** factor for magnification.

Answer 1226. Chemical

Frame 1227. Case hardening a lens can take as little as two minutes, where chemical hardening can require up to 18 hours.

An Optician who wishes to deliver a pair of glasses quickly then should resort to **(case hardening/chemical treating).**

Answer 813. 1.52

Frame 814. 1.52 will be thinner because the index of refraction is higher. The index of refraction of hilite is 1.69.

Because 1.69 is a higher number that 1.52 or 1.49, hilite must be the **(thickest/thinnest)** of the three.

Answer 951. three Who said this had to be hard?

Frame 952. Besides the "mirror" image clue of 1 2 4 5 6 7 8 8 9 9 8 8 7 6 5 4 2 1, this number is missing number 3.

Now, trust yourself. Cover the number in this frame and write it without looking.

Answer 1089. Power

Frame 1090. The total amount of magnification is the product of the shape factor and the power factor or $M_t = M_s \times M_p$ where

M_t = Total Magnification

M_s = Magnification due to shape ie. base curve and center thickness.

M_p = Vertex power from vertex distance.

The Optician first calculates the Shape Factor, then the Power Factor and **(divides/multiplies)** the two to obtain the total magnification.

Answer 1227. Case hardening

Frame 1228. The greatest advantage that chemical treating has over case hardening is that with case hardening the lenses cannot be safely re-shaped. Once the protective "case" is broken, as in re-edging, the impact resistance is weakened. Chemical treated lenses however, may be re-shaped without such consequences.

Therefore, the Optician who wishes the widest choice of lens management will use **(chemical/heat)** strengthening.

Answer 814. thinnest

Frame 815. Hilite (1.69) is the thinnest lens material for the Optician to choose from.*

So far, the law of opposites spoke only of thick and thin, but the law also holds true for weight.

The optical law of opposites include both thickness and **(wait/weight).**

*There are special indexes (indicies) that can be made, however.

Answer 952. 1 2 4 5 6 7 8 8 9 9 8 8 7 6 5 4 2 1

Frame 953. Once you have memorized the key number to oblique axis calculation, construct a chart similar to that illustrated in this frame: The chart lists the degrees away from the axis in **(5/10)** degree increments.

At ? degrees away from its axis	A cylinder has ? % of its power	At ? degrees away from its axis	A cylinder has ? % of its power
0-180		55-125	
5-175		60-120	
10-170		65-115	
15-165		70-110	
20-160		75-105	
25-155		80-100	
30-150		85- 95	
35-145		90- 90	
40-140		95- 85	
45-135		100- 80	
50-130			

Answer 1090. Multiplies.

Frame 1091. In more detail, the Shape Factor Formula is:

$$M_s = \frac{1}{1 - (\frac{t \times D}{n})}$$

Where: M_s = Shape Factor
t = Center Thickness in meters
n = index of refraction
D = Base Curve

Study the Rx in this frame and plug in the numbers. Check your answers in the next frame.

Rx O.D.	= +4.50
Base Curve	= +9.00
Thickness = 5.5 mm.	= .0055M
Index	= 1.523

Answer 1228. Chemical.

Frame 1229. In order to avoid inadvertently destroying a case-hardened lens, the Optician must be able to distinguish between the two types of strengthened lenses. A case-hardened lens will exhibit a particular shadow pattern when viewed between two pieces of poloroid material; a chemical-strengthened lens won't.

A shadow pattern **(can/can't)** distinguish a chemical-treated lens from a case-hardened lens.

Answer 815. Weight.

Frame 816. The higher the index (n), the heavier the lens. Test your knowledge of index of refraction in lens design by correctly matching the description in the columns below.

1) thickest — A. n = 1.69
2) thinnest — B. n = 1.52
3) heaviest — C. n = 1.49
4) lightest

Answer 953. 5.

Frame 954. The chart in Frame 953 lists cylinder axis in 5° increments. To find the percent of power for Column B of the chart, write the Key Number once again. Study the illustration in this frame. The illustration reproduces the chart and the correct **(Ki/Key)**.

Key 1 2 4 5 6 7 8 8 9 9 8 8 7 6 5 4 2 1

A AXIS	B % of Power	A AXIS	B % of Power
0-180	0	50-130	
5-175		55-125	
10-170		60-120	
15-165		65-115	
20-160		70-110	
25-155		75-105	
30-150		80-100	
35-145		85-95	
40-140		90-90	
45-135			

Answer 1091. Refer to Frame 1092.

Frame 1092.

$$M_s = \frac{1}{1 - \frac{(.0055 \times 9.00)}{1.523}} = 1.035 = 1.03\%.$$

Now for the Power Factor. The detailed formula for Power Factor (M_p) is: $M_p = \frac{1}{1 - (D_v \times h)}$

Where: M_p = Magnification due to Power
D_v = Lens power in diopters
h = Vertex distance (in meters)

This formula multiplies the lens power times the vertex distance in **(inches/meters)**.

Answer 1229. Can.

Frame 1230. Study the illustration in this frame. The illustration shows one type of instrument that Opticians use to view a strengthened lens through. The instrument is composed of two poloroid filters held by a common clasp to form a viewer.

Do you think this is called a **(polariscope/polarviewer)**?

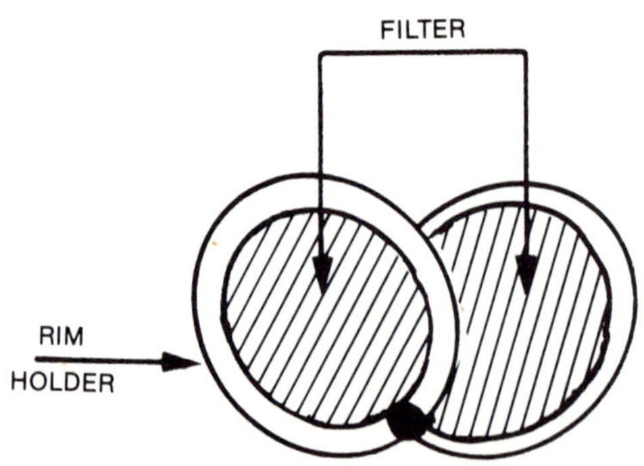

Answer 816. 1 C, 2 A, 3 A, 4 C.

Frame 817. In lens design, the Optician wisely selects the best lens material by understanding their consequences. For example, plastic will be light in weight but **(thin/thick).**

High index glass will be the thinnest but **(lightest/heaviest).**

Answer 954. Key.

Frame 955. Now, using the Key, calculate the percent of power a cylinder has. Begin adding one digit at a time and enter the result alongside the next proceeding axis. Study the example in this frame.

KEY 1 2 4 5 6 7 8 8 9 9 8 8 7 6 5 4 2 1

AXIS	% of Power	EXPLANATION
0-180	0	Step 1: Zero + 1 = 1
5-175	1	Step 2: 1 + 2 = 3
10-170	3	Step 3: 3 + 4 = 7
15-165	7	Step 4: 7 + 5 = 12
20-160	12	Step 5: 12 + 6 = 18
25-155	18	Step 6: 18 + 7 = 25
30-150	25	Step 7: 25 + 8 = 33
35-145	33	The next logical key
40-140	?	number to be added to
		33 would be **(8/9).**

Answer 1092. Meters.

Frame 1093. Study the power formula once again.

$$M_p = \frac{1}{1 - (D_v \times h)}$$

Now, calculate the magnification for the Rx +4.50 sphere as in Frame 1091 and check your answer in Frame 1094.

Vertex Distance = 13 mm. (h)
Power = 4.50 (D_v)

Answer 1230. Polariscope. (Some things have no logic!)

Frame 1231. The shadow pattern seen through a polariscope will vary somewhat from prescription to prescription. Study the shadow patterns illustrated in this frame.

The pattern that most resembles a Maltese cross is **(A/B/C)**.

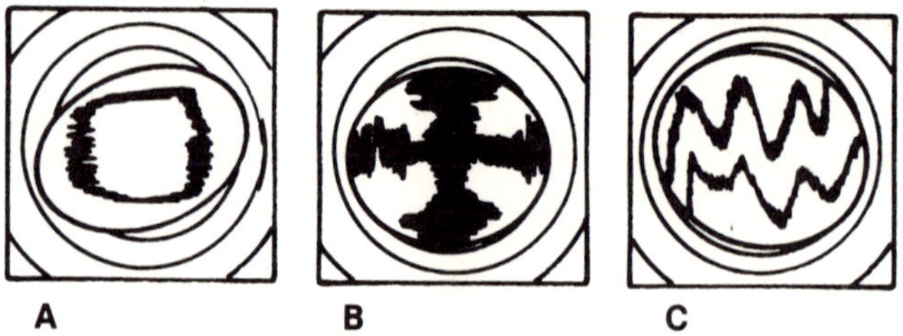

Answer 817. Thick, heaviest.

Frame 818. The best choice, of course, is directly dependent upon three factors: the wearer, the Rx, and how the prescription is to be used.

The integration of the above three factors, naturally, **(can/cannot)** affect patient satisfaction.

Answer 955. 8. (8 is next in line from the Key.)

Frame 956. Continue adding the next succeeding number from the Key to the last sum and enter it alongside your own chart until the chart is complete and looks like the one in this frame. The complete chart is found in Frame 957.

AXIS	% OF POWER	EXPLANATION
40-140	41	Step 8: 33 + 8 = 41
45-135	50	Step 9: 41 + 9 = 50
50-130	59	Step 10: 50 + 9 = 59
55-125	67	Step 11: 59 + 8 = 67
60-120	75	Step 12: 67 + 8 = 75
65-115	82	Step 13: 75 + 7 = 82
70-110	88	Step 14: 82 + 6 = 88
75-105	93	Step 15: 88 + 5 = 93
80-100	97	Step 16: 93 + 4 = 97
85- 95	99	Step 17: 97 + 2 = 99
90- 90	100	Step 18: 99 + 1 = 100

Answer 1093. None required. Please continue.

Frame 1094.

$$M_p = \frac{1}{1 - (D_v \times h)}$$

$$M_p = \frac{1}{1 - (+4.50 \times .013)}$$

$$M_p = \frac{1}{1 - (.0585)}$$

$$M_p = \frac{1}{.9415}$$

$$M_p = 1.062$$

The magnification formula states: Total magnification is the product of shape factor (M_s) times Power Factor (M_p). The Optician must **(multiply/divide)**.

Answer 1231. B.

Frame 1232. The polariscope shadow pattern distinguishes the case-hardened or heat-treated lens from the chemical-treated lens. Test your understanding of this Chapter by correctly matching the descriptions in Column B with the characteristics in Column A. (You may choose more than one.)

COLUMN A	COLUMN B
1. Takes 15 hours or more to process.	A. Industrial Safety
2. Shows a shadow pattern through a polariscope.	B. Chemical Treated
3. Takes minutes to process.	C. Heat Treated
4. Can be re-shaped.	D. Case Hardened
5. Requires a 3 mm. thickness.	E. Street Safety
6. Requires dropball test only.	

Answer 818. Can. Naturally!

Frame 819. As stated earlier, lens design is affected by prescription, base curve, lens material and size.

Consider a minus lens. Because the edges are thicker than the center, the larger the lens size, the thicker the edge becomes.

Study the illustration in this frame. The illustration shows two lenses of the same power, but different sizes. Lens **(A/B)** has thicker edges because it is **(larger/smaller)**.

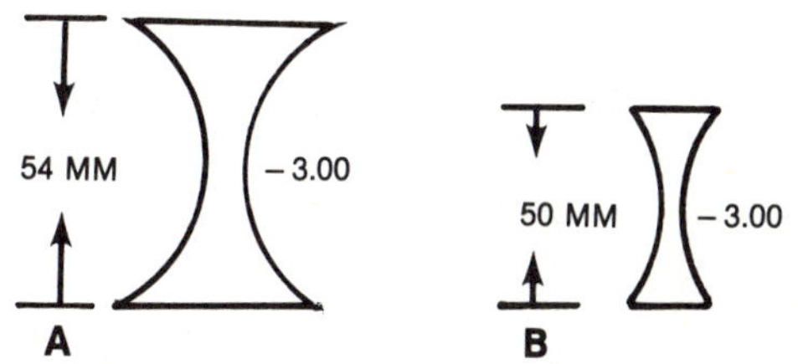

Answer 956. None required.

Frame 957. Compare your chart with the complete one represented here and turn to the next frame, number 958.

Key 1 2 4 5 6 7 8 8 9 9 8 8 7 6 5 4 2 1

AXIS	% OF POWER	AXIS	% OF POWER
0-180	0	50-130	59
5-175	1	55-125	67
10-170	3	60-120	75
15-165	7	65-115	82
20-160	12	70-110	88
25-155	18	75-105	93
30-150	25	80-100	97
35-145	33	85-95	99
40-140	41	90-90	100
45-135	50		

Answer 1094. Multiply.

Frame 1095. The Shape Factor M_s × the Power Factor M_p equals the total magnification (M_t). For the Rx +4.50 the M_s was 1.035 and the M_p was 1.062. Therefore:

$M_t = M_s \times M_p$
$M_t = 1.035 \times 1.062$
$M_t = 1.099$ or 9.9% magnification O.D.

Study the Rx in this frame.

O.D. +4.50 sph
O.S. +1.00 sph

The Rx reproduces the same O.D. as in Frame 1091. The O.S. is +1.00 sph. Do you think the magnification difference between O.D. and O.S. will cause problems? **(Yes/No)**

Answer 1232. 1) B, 2) C & D, 3) C & E, 4) B, 5) A, 6) E.

Frame 1233.

CHAPTER 22
INSPECTION

TURN TO THE BOTTOM OF PAGE 128, **FRAME 1234**

Answer 819. A, larger.

Frame 820. The larger lens size has the thicker edge. Opticians, then, who wish to avoid excess thickness, will choose **(smaller/larger)** eye sizes.

One factor that accompanies lens size is decentration. Usually, the frame P.D. is greater than the patient's P.D., therefore resulting in decentration **(nasal/temporal).**

Answer 957. None required. (You are doing very well!)

Frame 958. You now have a very workable chart which allows for the calculation of the percent of power a cylinder will have as it moves away from its axis. Some cylinder power calculation can be deduced and this makes use of the chart even easier.

For example: A cylinder has **(0/100)** percent of its power at its axis.

Answer 1095. Yes. (Let's see why.)

Frame 1096. This frame contains the data for magnification for the O.S.

O.S. +1.00 sph

t = 2.5 mm. = .0025 M
n = 1.523
D = Base Curve +6.00
D_v = +1.00 sph
h = 13 mm. = .0013 M

Calculate the total magnification and check your answer in Frame 1097.

Answer 1233. None required.

Frame 1234. The Optician has the job of inspecting the finished glasses to see if they are exactly as ordered. The most efficient way to accomplish this is to establish a routine in which the order of inspection and verification becomes habit. Study the list of a partial routine in this frame.

1. Frame Color
2. Size
3. Style
4. Model Number
5. Etc.

Standardized routines help the Optician keep track of the many facets of **(verification/prevarication)**.

Answer 820. Smaller, nasal.

Frame 821. Decentration will affect lens design by placing the thicker portion of a lens toward the nose in a **(plus/minus)** lens and toward the temple in a **(minus/plus)** lens.

Decentration may also be vertical, thus affecting the lens at its top and **(bottom/sides)**.

Answer 958. 0 (zero percent).

Frame 959. A cylinder has 100% of its power at 90° from its axis. Take a moment to review what you already know. Study the example in this frame and complete the chart.

Rx	Power 90° From Axis	0 or 180° From Axis
Ex) + 3.00 × 90	+3.00	0
A) +4.00 × 180	?	?
B) −6.00 × 175	?	?
C) −2.50 × 130	?	?
D) +10.00 × 45	?	?

Answer 1096. Go to Frame 1097.

Frame 1097. O.S. +1.00 sph

$$M_s = \frac{1}{1-(\frac{t \times D}{n})} = \frac{1}{1-(\frac{.0025 \times 6.00}{1.523})} = 1.001$$

$$M_p = \frac{1}{1-(D_v \times h)} = \frac{1}{1-(+1.00 \times .013)} = 1.013$$

$$M_t = M_s \times M_p = 1.001 \times 1.013 = 1.014 = 1.4\%$$

Look back at your answer for total magnification for the O.D. = 9.9%. The difference in magnification, then, between O.D. and O.S. is 9.9 − 1.4 or = 8.5%.

The O.D. sees an image 8.5% **(larger/smaller)** than the O.S.

Answer 1234. Verification.

Frame 1235. Standardization of inspection methods work very well for frames, but since Optical meridians may vary, the Rx verification **(can/cannot)** be committed to standardization. If the right eye is always checked in the lensometer first, for instance, and then the left eye, the Optician may encounter induced prism. Study the Rx in this frame.

O.D. −0.50 +0.50 × 180
O.S. −4.00 sph

The vertical meridian O.D. is **(+0.50/Plano)**.

Answer 821. **Plus, minus, bottom.**

Frame 822. Plus lenses have thicker centers than edges. They also have another factor: Magnification.

Decentration causing the thickest portion of the lens to be moved nasally, for example, will **(minify/magnify)** that area.

Answer 959. **A) +4.00 × 90, 0.00 × 180** **B) −6.00 × 85, 0.00 × 175**
C) −2.50 × 40, 0.00 × 130 **D) +10.00 × 135, 0.00 × 45**

Frame 960. All cylinders have none of their power at their axes; that is, 0 or 180° from their axes. All cylinders have all or 100% of their power at 90° from their axes. After all, isn't that what cylinders are? **(Yes/No).**

If a cylinder has all of its power at 90° from its axis, do you suppose at 45°, or halfway, from its axis it will have **(50/75)** percent?

Answer 1097. Larger.

Frame 1098. The Optician can compensate for magnification through the use of base curve, thickness, and vertex distance. For example, increasing the base curve will increase the image size. Study the two base curves in this frame.

The base curve which will increase the image size and therefore create more magnification is **(A/B).**

A) +3.00 sph. Base Curve +10.00
B) +3.00 sph. Base Curve + 6.00

Answer 1235. Cannot, Plano.

Frame 1236. The position of the center in a Plano lens can establish a false vertical height so that the O.S. lens will appear to sit with its center higher or lower in comparison. Study the example in this frame. The example illustrates a view through the lensometer at two Rx's.

This Rx now appears to have **(vertical/horizontal)** imbalance.

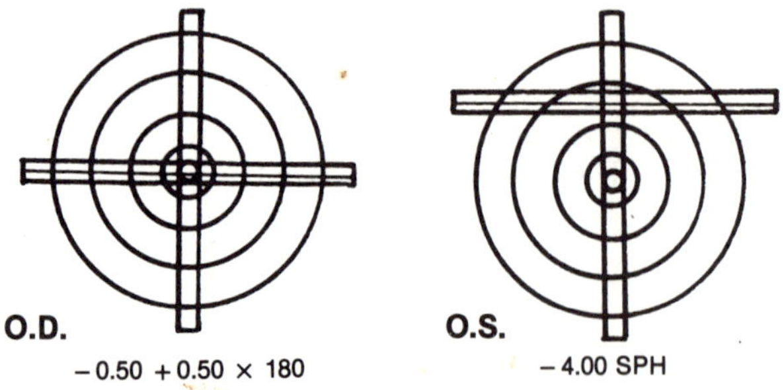

Answer 822. Magnify.

Frame 823. Exactly how much magnification occurs as a result of decentration depends upon the lens power, the amount of decentration, and the lens material itself. The subject of magnification will be discussed in another chapter. Test your knowledge of basic lens design by correctly matching the answers in Column A with those in Column B.

COLUMN A	COLUMN B
a. high index	1. Thinnest lens
b. no decentration	2. Thickest lens
c. smaller vs. larger size	
d. lab recommended curves	
e. low index	
f. decentration	
g. larger vs. smaller size	

Answer 960. Yes — 50% (of course)!

Frame 961. You will need your chart* for reference as you work the next series of frames. Look at the chart once again. Opticians are mostly interested in significant changes which may influence patients and their prescriptions.

A cylinder power of 1 to 7% is generally considered **(significant/insignificant).**

*An easy-to-read full chart can be found in the Appendix, page 278.

Answer 1098. A.

Frame 1099. The higher the base curve, the greater the magnification will be. Increasing the lens thickness will increase the magnification also. Study the examples in this frame.

The lens which will have the most magnification is **(A/B/C).**

A) −2.00 Center Thickness 2.0 mm.
B) −2.00 Center Thickness 3.3 mm.
C) −2.00 Center Thickness 5.0 mm.

Answer 1236. Vertical.

Frame 1237. Failure to analyze the Rx about to be inspected through the lensometer, can cause the Optician to misread the finished prescriptions.

Think about the last example once again. If the Optician had centered and read the O.S. first, then vertical imbalance would **(have not/still have)** been observed.

Answer 823. **a1, b1, c1, d1 — e2, f2, g2.**

Frame 824.

CHAPTER 4
LENS ABNORMALITIES

CONTINUE ON TO **FRAME 825**, ON THE TOP OF PAGE 137
(NOT A HARD CHAPTER)

Answer 961. **Insignificant.**

Frame 962. Except for super strong cylinder powers, Opticians can generally ignore the small 1-7% of a given power. For example: 7% of a 5.00 cylinder is only .35 D or a fraction more than 1/3 of a diopter! Consider the other end of the chart for a moment. A cylinder which has at least 80% of its power can really be considered to have most of its power.

You see, the chart has now become considerably **(smaller/larger)**.

Answer 1099. C.

Frame 1100. Both Base Curve and Center Thickness can be used to increase magnification. Study the Rx's in this frame.

O.D. −4.00 sph
O.S. −0.75 sph

The magnification of the O.S. **(can/cannot)** be increased by using a +8.00 base and 3.5 center thickness rather than a +6.00 base and a 2.2 center thickness.

Answer 1237. Have not.

Frame 1238. The following routine can guide the Optician to Rx inspection and verification. The routine consists of four guidelines.

The First Guideline

1. The Optician should always first verify any lens with prescription power before a lens without power.

Study the Rx in this frame. The lens which should be verified is **(O.D./O.S.)**.

O.D. Plano
O.S. +2.00

Answer 824. No answer needed. Go to Frame 825.

Frame 825. The dispensing Optician has control over lens design in the sense there is control over the choice of curves, material, size, and decentration. Lenses, however, must also be inherently free from lens abnormalities.

A well-designed lens must be free from lens **(abnormalities/aborigionies)**.

Answer 962. Smaller.

Frame 963. If you only memorized the remainder of the chart, that is, the center section, consisting of ten items, you would have a good handle on calculating oblique axis problems. Here is how the chart is used.

Problem: What is the power of a −4.00 cylinder whose axis is 135, at axis 180? *Or* −4.00 × 135 =? × 180.

Solution: Step 1: 135 is **(45/90)** from 180? (How many degrees away from the given axis is the wanted meridian?)

Answer 1100. Can.

. . . .

Frame 1101. The third tool for the Optician in control of magnification is Vertex Distance. In Plus lenses, increasing the vertex distance will increase the magnification. Study the illustration in this frame. The illustration shows two vertex distances.

Vertex distance **(A/B)** has the greatest magnification.

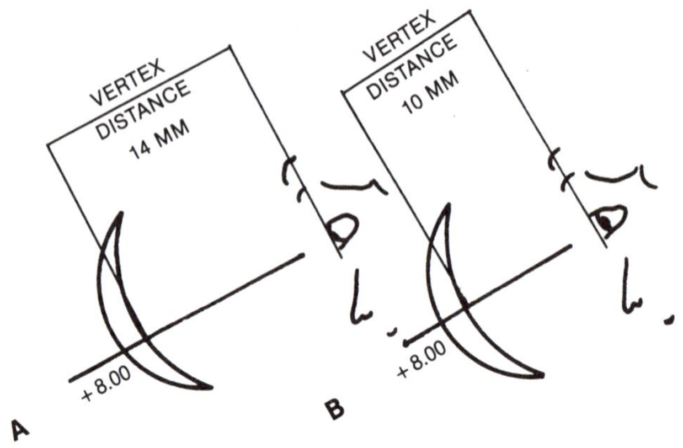

Answer 1238. O.S.

. . . .

Frame 1239. The second guideline.

2. Is to verify the stronger of any two plano cylinders first. Study the Rx's in this frame. Select the lens which are to be verified first. **(A, O.D./O.S.) (B, O.D./O.S.)**.

A) O.D. Plano +1.00 × 180
O. S. Plano +0.75 × 90

B) O.D. Plano −0.75 × 165
O. S. Plano −2.75 × 75

Answer 825. Abnormalities.

Frame 826. Lens abnormalities can occur during the manufacturing process. Some of these abnormalities include pits, scratches, strae, waves, and aberrations. Such abnormalities are rejected at the manufacturing site as undesirable as a first quality lens.

These lenses may, however, be sold as **(first/second)** quality lenses.

Answer 963. 45.

Frame 964. Axis 135 is 45 degrees away from 180.

Step 2: Looking at your chart, under Column A, "Degrees away from axis," 45 is found on the 45-135 line and the percent of power reads **(145/50)** %.

Answer 1101. A.

Frame 1102. Increasing the vertex distance in plus lenses also increases magnification. Minus lenses are opposite of plus, therefore, increasing the vertex distance of minus lenses decreases magnification. Complete the chart in this frame to demonstrate your understanding of the vertex distance role in magnification.

Power	Moved From	VD mm.	to	VD mm.	=	increases yes / no	decreases magnification yes / no
Example: − 6.00		10mm.		15mm.		no	yes
A) +10.00		13		15		?	?
B) − 4.00		12		8		?	?
C) + 7.50		14		9		?	?
D) − 8.00		11		14		?	?

Answer 1239. A, O.D. B, O.S.

Frame 1240. The third guideline.

3. Is to verify any compound lens first, before any plano cylinder.

Which do you think is the correct lens to verify first in the examples below?

A) O.D. +2.75 +1.75 × 45
O.S. Plano +1.75 × 135

B) O.D. Plano +2.50 × 90
O.S. −2.50 +3.50 × 180

Answer 826. second

Frame 827. Lenses that fail to pass strict inspection are labeled "seconds" and sold to outlets who have less demanding standards.

Because the market may contain lenses of less than first quality, the dispensing Optician must be alert to the **(quantity/quality)** of the lenses used.

Answer 964. 50%

Frame 965. At 45 or 135 degrees away from its axis then, a cylinder has 50% of its power. For the problem in Frame 963. A −4.00 × 135 has 50% of its power, or −2.00, in the 180 meridian. Try another one.

PROBLEM: Rx +6.00 × 150 should have been decentered up 4 mm. What prismatic effect has this caused?

SOLUTION: Since decentration up and down is considered; the meridian in question, will be **(90/180).**

Answer 1102. A — increases, B — increases, C — decreases, D — decreases.

Frame 1103. Base curve, lens center thickness and vertex distance all influence magnification. The Optician must decide whether to increase or decrease magnification in the attempt to balance aniseikonic prescriptions. Study the reproduction of Rx and data for Frames 1091 and 1096. Once again, this Rx **(is/is not)** aniseikonic.

EYE POWER	BASE CURVE	THICKNESS	VERTEX DISTANCE
O.D. +4.50	+6.00	2.5 mm.	13 mm.
O.S. +1.00	+9.50	5.5 mm.	13 mm.

____

Answer 1240. (A) O.D., (B) O.S.

Frame 1241. The fourth guideline

4. Is to verify the stronger of any two spheres or any two compound lenses first.

Study the Rx's below and choose the correct lenses to verify first.

A) O.D. +6.00 sph
O.S. +5.75 sph

B) O.D. −4.00 +2.00 × 60
O.S. −3.75 +2.00 × 150

C) O.D. +12.00 −3.75 × 180
O.S. +15.00 −2.00 × 180

D) O.D. −1.00 sph
O.S. −0.50 sph

____

Answer 827. Quality.

Frame 828. Lenses can have other abnormalities called aberrations. Lens aberrations are negative optical characteristics which occur as light passes through a lens with some particular combination of curves, index of refraction, and thickness.

Some lens abnormalities are **(positive/negative)** optical characteristics which can be called **(habitations/aberrations).**

Answer 965. 90.

Frame 966. Solution (continued) . . .

Step 1: 90 is how many degrees away from 150? (150 − 90 = 60)
90 is 60° away from axis 150.

Step 2: At 60-120 degrees away from its axis, a cylinder has 75% of its power (consult chart).

Step 3: 75% of +6.00 = 4.50.
The Rx +6.00 × 150 has +4.50 of power at axis 90.

Step 4: Failure to decenter +4.50 4 mm. =

$$\Delta = \frac{d \times P}{10} = \frac{4 \times \mathbf{(4.50/6.00)}}{10}$$

Answer 1103. Is.

Frame 1104. The Optician must increase magnification of the O.S. and decrease the magnification of the O.D. to balance the aniseikonia.

This would be most correctly illustrated by situation **(A/B)**.

	EYE POWER	BASE CURVE	THICKNESS	VERTEX DISTANCE
A)	O.D. +4.50 O.S. +1.00	+9.50 +6.00	5.5 mm. 2.5 mm.	13 mm. 13 mm.
B)	O.D. +4.50 O.S. +1.00	+6.00 +10.00	4.0 mm. 4.0 mm.	16 mm. 11 mm.

Answer 1241. (A) O.D., (B) O.D., (C) O.S., (D) O.D.

Frame 1242. When oblique axis are involved the Optician must consider the combined prismatic effect which may be viewed through the lensometer as the lenses are placed from one position to another. See Frames 997, 998.

When analyzing the prescription for inspection and verification the Optician must be very alert to powers and oblique meridians **(differences/equality)**.

Answer 828. negative, aberrations

Frame 829. Lens aberrations can be identified into categories. One such category deals with the phenomonon of light breaking into its individual color components (rainbow) as it passes through a prism. The scientific word for color is "chroma".

Therefore, the aberration could be called **(chromatic/chorodial)** aberration.

Answer 966. $\Delta = \dfrac{4 \times 4.50}{10} = 1.8$

Frame 967. Failure to vertically decenter a +6.00 × 1.50 4 mm. results in a 1.8 Δ prismatic effect. Since the solution to oblique axis problems are multi-step, a very carefully prepared procedure will lead to success and avoid confusion

In order to solve multi-step problems the Optician must develope a prepared **(plan/plane)**.

Answer 1104. B

Frame 1105. The preceeding Rx B can compensate for the aniseikonia in Rx A by reducing the total magnification from 8.5% to a mere 2.5%. In general, the most successful Rx's to compensate are those with less than 5% magnification difference, that is, one with four or less diopters of difference between O.D. and O.S.

Which Rx do you think would be the most successful if attempted to balance, **(A/B)**?

A) O.D. +8.00
O.S. +1.50

B) O.D. +4.75
O.S. +0.50

Answer 1242. Differences

Frame 1243. Sometimes the stronger of two Rx's is difficult to ascertain. Study the Rx's in this frame.

O.D. +1.75 −3.00 × 90
O.S. +2.00 −2.50 × 180

Which eye do you think is stronger, **(O.D./O.S.)**?

Answer 829. **Chromatic.**

Frame 830. Chromatic aberration is one category of aberration. Another form occurs as light bends unevenly around the very edges or margins of the lens.

Do you think this category of aberration is called **(magical/marginal)** aberration?

Answer 967. **Plan. "If you don't know where you're going, chances are you will wind up somewhere else."**

Frame 968. Test yourself on oblique cylinder analysis by correctly completing the chart below.

Rx	Power at 90	Power at 180
Ex) +4.00 × 30	+3.00	+1.00
A) −2.00 × 45	?	?
B) +1.00 × 60	?	?
C) −3.25 × 135	?	?

Answer 1105. B.

Frame 1106. It is better to alter base curve and vertex distance rather than thickness in myopes. In Hyperopes, it is better to alter lens thickness and vertex distance rather than base curve. Study the chart in this frame and choose the correct response, based upon the above statement.

	CHANGE BASE CURVE	THICKNESS	VERTEX DISTANCE
A) IN MINUS	**(Yes/No)**	**(Yes/No)**	**(Yes/No)**
B) IN PLUS	**(Yes/No)**	**(Yes/No)**	**(Yes/No)**

Answer 1243. O.S. Let's see why!

Frame 1244. One way to determine the difference in strength between two eyes is to reduce the Rx to spherical equivalents. As you will remember, the spherical equivalent is found by adding one-half (50%) of the cylinder power to the sphere power.

Look at the Rx's in 1243 once again.

Spherical Equivalent = O.D. +1.75 −3.00 × 90
= (+1.75) + (−1.50) = +0.25

Spherical Equivalent = O.S. +2.00 −2.50 × 180
= (+2.00) + (−1.25) = +0.75

Which is stronger? **(+0.75/+0.25)** Which lens should be inspected first? **(O.D./O.S.)**

Answer 830. Marginal; told you this was not hard!

Frame 831. Some aberrations create cylinders as a result of the way light passes through a lens. This type of aberration is called **(astigmatic/automatic)** aberration.

Coma, curvature of field, and distortion are some of the other aberrations that have been identified.

Answer 968.

A)	B)	C)
−1.00 × 180	**+0.25 × 90**	**−1.62 × 90**
−1.00 × 90	**+0.75 × 180**	**−1.62 × 180**

Frame 969.

CHAPTER 12
SPHERO-CYLINDER ANALYSIS

TURN TO THE BOTTOM OF PAGE 151, **FRAME 970**

Answe 1106. A) Yes — No — Yes B) No — Yes — Yes.

Frame 1107. Because compensating for aniseikonia requires altering the prescription from the ordinary, it is important to first assess the chances for success. Information such as how well both eyes work together, and the stability of the new Rx is the Doctor's domain. It would be wise, therefore, to **(confer/ignore)** the Doctor before undertaking drastic changes in prescription parameters.

Answer 1244. +0.75, O.S.

Frame 1245. When the axis of two compound lenses are symmetrical, that is, 90° apart, then the spherical equivalent is easy to calculate. When the axis is asymmetrical, the spherical equivalent is calculated the same way as symmetrical axis, but the determination of the "difference" in power between the two eyes requires the mathematics of geometry and trigonometry.

Study the Rx in this frame.

O.D. +2.00 +1.75 × 20
O.S. +1.50 +2.50 × 150

The spherical equivalent of this Rx is O.D. **(+3.75/+2.87)** and O.S. **(+1.25/+2.75)**.

Answer 831. Astigmatic.

Frame 832. Distortion aberration is divided into two categories: Barrel Distortion, and Pincushion Distortion. Study the diagrams in this frame. The diagrams illustrate two types of distortion.

Which do you think is an example of Barrel Distortion? **(A/B)**

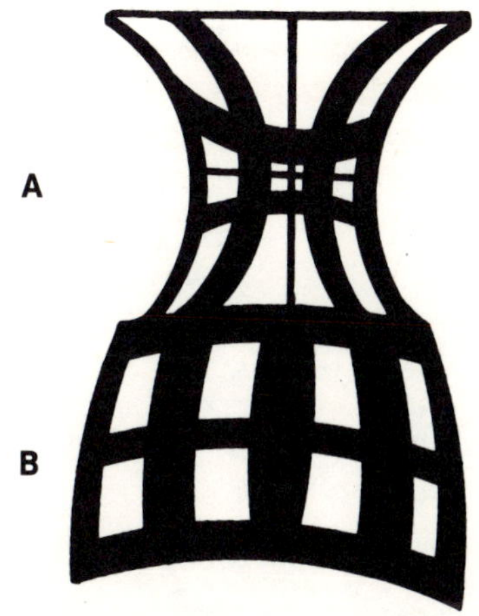

Answer 969. None required.

Frame 970. Spherocylindrical analysis allows the Optician to calculate the *total* lens power of any Rx in any given meridian.

Chapter 11 dealt with analysis of the cylinder component only, however, when the spherical element is added, the total power may **(change/remain unchanged)**.

Answer 1107. Confer.

Frame 1108. The decision to compensate is not so much "where" as "when." The password should be 'caution.' It's a little like the difference between wisdom and knowledge; knowledge is knowing exactly what to do . . . and wisdom is knowing **(when/when not)** to do it!

____

Answer 1245. +2.87, +2.75.

Frame 1246. The spherical equivalents will help the Optician find the stronger of any two compound lenses, but in order to find the difference in power when the axis is non-symmetrical, the Optician must use **(higher/lower)** mathematics.

____

Answer 832. B.

Frame 833. Barrel distortion causes objects to appear Barrel-like or bowed out. Pincushion distortion causes objects to appear curved inward.

If a patient reported that the doorway curved inward, the Optician may suspect **(barrel/pincushion)** distortion.

Answer 970. Change.

Frame 971. The addition of the spherical element can drastically change the total lens power in a given meridian. Study the example in this frame.

Rx −2.50 +5.00 × 45

The power of the cylinder only at axis 180 is +2.50 and the power of the sphere at axis 180 is **(−2.50/+5.00)**.

Answer 1108. When not. (You bet!)

Frame 1109.

CHAPTER 16
VERTEX DISTANCE

TURN TO THE TOP OF PAGE 156, **FRAME 1110**

Answer 1246. Higher.

Frame 1247.

CHAPTER 23
THE DEADLY Rx

TURN TO THE BOTTOM OF PAGE 156, **FRAME 1248**

Answer 833. Pincushion.

Frame 834. Some distortions can be induced, that is, created during the surfacing or finishing process. A plastic lens which is mounted under excessive pressure, for example, may warp, thus creating **(this torsion/distortion).**

Answer 971. −2.50 (A sphere has equal power in all meridians.)

Frame 972. The addition of the spherical component of Rx −2.50 +5.00 × 45 to the cylinder power at axis 180 is illustrated in this frame.

Power of +5.00 cylinder axis 45 at 180	=	+2.50
Power of −2.50 sphere at 180	=	−2.50
TOTAL POWER OF LENS AT 180	=	0.00

The Rx −2.50 +5.00 × 45 in the horizontal meridian of 180 is PLANO!

If you placed the Rx −2.50 +5.00 × 45 in the lensometer and rotated the axis wheel to 180, the reading would **(−2.50/+5.00/0.00).**

Answer 1109. None required.

Frame 1110. When the vertex distance of a prescription changes, the effective power of the prescription also changes. Plus lenses become stronger and minus lenses become weaker as they increase their vertex distances.

Since their lens power is directly related to focal length, the secret to vertex distance compensation concerns **(focal/facial)** length.

Answer 1247. None required.

Frame 1248. As you have seen by studying the Chapters so far, the Optician must keep alert to many things when it comes to Rx's. As often happens, when alertness is at a low level, problems can occur. This can cause the Optician time, money, unhappy Doctors, and dissatisfied patients. When this does happen, it is as if the Rx has 'turned' upon you.

That is why this author calls it the **(deadly/doozy)** Rx.

Answer 834. distortion

Frame 835. Lens aberrations are of special in terest to the optical scientist as he trys to create the perfect lens.

The dispensing Optician must understand that there is no perfect lens and that all lenses have some form of aberration.

The dispenser should try to avoid these aberrations by using only the best designed and quality controlled lenses available while understanding that there is **(one/no)** perfect lens.

Answer 972. 0.00

Frame 973. As a dispensing Optician you can utilize spherocylinder analysis to compute decentration, prism, or E.D. Follow the steps in the example illustrated in this frame.

Example: +1.75 −3.50 × 135 2 Δ BI

Question: Can prism be achieved thru decentration or must prism be ordered from the lab?

Answer: Step 1 - What is the cylinder power × 180?
Step 2 - What is the sphere power × 180?
Step 3 - What is the needed decentration?

Work your answer and compare with the solution in Frame 974.

Answer 1110. Focal.

Frame 1111. Opticians use the focal length formula: $f = \frac{1000}{D}$ to find the focal length of a lens when the dioptric power is known. Study the formula in this frame.

$$f = \frac{1000}{D}$$

where f = focal length
D = lens power in Diopters

Find the focal length of the following Rx's:
A) +9.00 B) −6.00

Unless you enjoy long division by hand, get your calculator and I'll meet you in the next frame with the answers.

Answer 1248. Deadly.

Frame 1249. This Deadly Rx Chapter is a series of collected examples: Prescriptions and situations which point out the value of remaining alert. If you are ready, then so am I. (This Chapter requires all the knowledge of the previous Chapters.)

Title: **THE BUMS RUSH**

Situation: It is lunch time and everyone but you is out. A patient arrives, rushed, stating that he must leave town and needs his glasses quick. You show and sell a tasteful goggle frame. You check your stock drawer and find 65 mm. blanks.

Data: Rx O.D. −1.50 +3.00 × 135
O. S. −1.00 +2.00 × 45
P.D. 60
52/20 Goggle Shape
E.D. 54

Question: Does this Rx need oversize? **(Yes/No)** Or can you use 65 mm. and get the job on time? **(Yes/No)**

Answer 835. **No.**

Frame 836.

CHAPTER 5
THE CROSSED CYLINDER

TURN TO THE TOP OF PAGE 161, **FRAME 837**

Answer 973. **See Frame 974.**

Frame 974. Answer to Frame 973 is found in this frame.

Step 1: 135 is 45 degrees from 180.

Step 2: At 45 or 135 degrees from its axis a cylinder has 50% of its power.

Step 3: 50% of the cylinder −3.50 = −1.75.

Step 4: +1.75 sphere has +1.75 power × 180.

Step 5: (+1.75) + (−1.75) = 0.00

Step 6: $d = \frac{10 \times \Delta}{P}$

Step 7: $d = \frac{10 \times 2}{0.00} = \frac{20}{0} = 0$

Conclusion: Since the total power at 180 is 0.00, no decentration is possible and if Δ is to be achieved, it must be sent to the **(lab/lap)**.

Answer 1111. None required for now. (We'll get you later.)

Frame 1112.. $f = \frac{1000}{D}$

A) $f = \frac{1000}{+9.00} = +111$ mm.

B) $f = \frac{1000}{-6.00} = -166$ mm.

When Dioptric Power is needed, the Optician uses the formula $D = \frac{1000}{f}$.

Find the power of the lenses in this frame.

1. Lens B has a negative focal length of −166 mm.
2. Lens A has a positive focal length of one-hundred-eleven millimeters.

Answer 1249. No, Yes. Let's see why.

Frame 1250. *Question No. 1:* Does this Rx require oversize?

Solution: Optician needs to know needed lens blank size.

Calculation:

[('A' Box+Dbl) − (P.D.)] + 54 = NLBS
[52+20) − (60)] + 54 = NLBS
[(72) − (60)] + 54 = NLBS
12 + 54 = NLBS
66 = NLBS

If standard blank size is 65 mm., then oversize is theoretically required, but. . .

Question No. 2: What is the consequence of not decentering 1 mm.?

Calculation: $\text{O.D.} = \Delta = \frac{d \times P}{10} = \frac{(1) \times (0)^*}{10} = 0$

$\text{O.S.} = \Delta = \frac{d \times P}{10} = \frac{1 \times 0}{10} = 0$

*Horizontal meridian has **(some/no)** power.

Answer 836. Go to Frame 837.

Frame 837. Chapter Three spoke of plus or minus cylinder lens design from which the dispensing Optician may choose. Another choice exists, however, where the lens design is one in which a cylinder may be ground on both front **and** back surfaces; the crossed cylinder.

The Optician may design a lens in minus, plus and **(crossed/christ)** cylinders.

Answer 974. lab

Frame 975. The ability to analyze any given Rx in the horizontal and vertical meridians allows the dispenser to understand the role of decentration, better control costs for larger lens sizes, and predict possible problem areas. Chapters Ten and Eleven dealt with the role of decentration, prism, as well as needed lens blank size.

The subject of predicting possible problem **(areas/arias)** continues with Frame 976.

Answer 1112. 1) $D = \frac{1000}{f} = \frac{1000}{-166} = -6.00$ 2) $D = \frac{1000}{f} = \frac{1000}{111} = +9.00$

Frame 1113. The effective power of lenses changes very little with lower power lenses, however, the effective power change can be significant. Consider a +5.00 sphere. Suppose this patient was wearing a frame with adjustable nose pads and the vertex distance was 14 mm. While on a trip, the frame was broken and replaced with one without adjustable pads. This caused the lens to sit closer to the face with a new vertex distance of 8 mm. Do you think the effective power of this lens will now be **(greater than/less than)** +5.00?

Answer 1250. **No**

Frame 1251. COMMENT: Because decentration for P.D. occurs at 180° and no power exists at 180, no prism horizontally will be created if the Optician fails to decenter.

Prism **will** be created, however, vertically (see Chapter Twelve, Frames 997-998), but, with only a couple of millimeters of decentration and the given power of this Rx, it will be minimal and well within allowances.

The Optician who merely looks at the Rx without analyzing the meridians may lose the sale and the **(patient/patent)**.

Answer 837. crossed

Frame 838. Study the illustration in this frame. The illustration shows a **(−2.00 +1.00 × 180/−1.00 −1.00 × 090/either)**

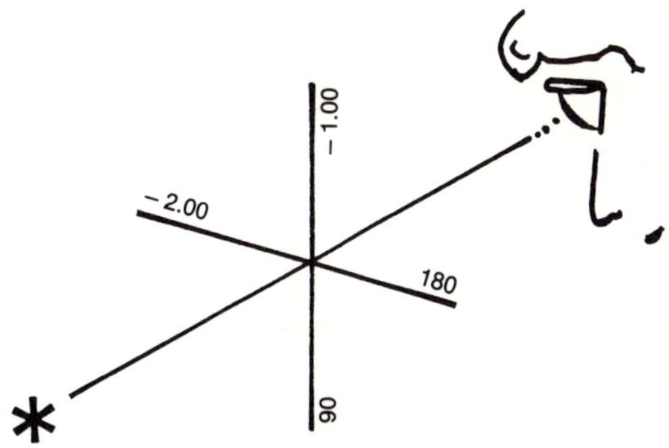

Answer 975. areas

Frame 976. Study the Rx in this frame.

+2.00 +1.00 × 90

Mentally picture this lens directly in front of your left eye. As you look out, this lens has **(+2.00/+3.00)** vertically and **(+1.00/+3.00)** horizontally. Since your line of sight passes directly through the optical center of this lens, there is **(some/no)** prismatic effect.

Answer 1113. Less than

Frame 1114. Study the diagram in this frame. The diagram illustrates a +5.00 sph in each situation with a vertex distance of 14 mm. in example A and a vertex distance of **(8 mm./6 mm.)** in example B.

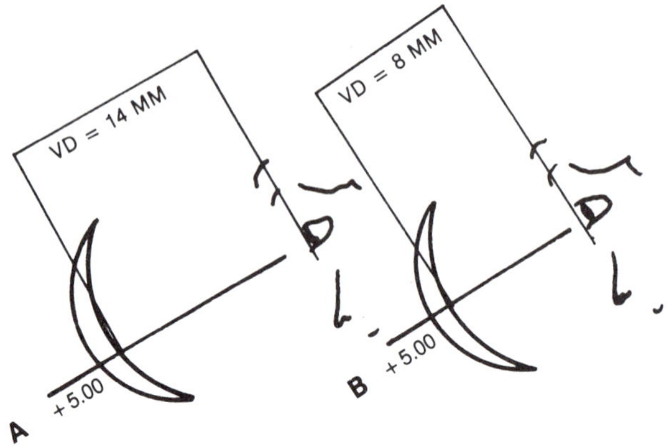

Answer 1251. Patient

Frame 1252.

Title: **VERIFICATION**

Situation: It is a very busy day and the Optician doing check out manages to catch you between patients. You are told that the Rx is 5 mm. off P.D. and Mrs. Finn E. Key just called checking on the job. Being a conscientious dispenser, you say "The job has got to be right" and scurry off to your next patient. The check out Optician returns the Rx to the lab with giant red pen script pointing out the P.D. error. The lab checks the job and finds it within tolerance, but cannot get through to your telephone line.

Answer 838. Either.

Frame 839. The illustration in Frame 838 is read in minus cylinder as −1.00 −1.00 × 090 and in plus cylinder as −2.00 +1.00 × 180. By combining the opposite axis with the power in a given meridian, the crossed cylinder form may be found. Follow this example.

If the 090 axis is chosen in Frame 838, the power in that meridian is **(−2.00/−1.00)**.

Answer 976. +2.00, +3.00, No.

Frame 977. Continue with the mental image of +2.00 +1.00 × 90 in front of your left eye. As your eye travels downwards to read, it **(is/is not)** moving away from the optical center. If it moves a distance of 8 mm. it is as if the lens had been decentered **(downward/upward)** thus **(creating/negating)** a prismatic effect of:

$$\Delta = \frac{d \times P}{10} = \frac{8 \times 2.00}{10} = 1.6$$

Answer 1114. 8 mm.

Frame 1115. This frame reproduces the same example as in Frame 1114. The examples now have dotted lines added representing focal length. From visual inspection alone, you can see that the focus of example A is on the retina as it should be. However, because the lens has been brought closer, the focus in example B is **(in front of/behind)** the retina.

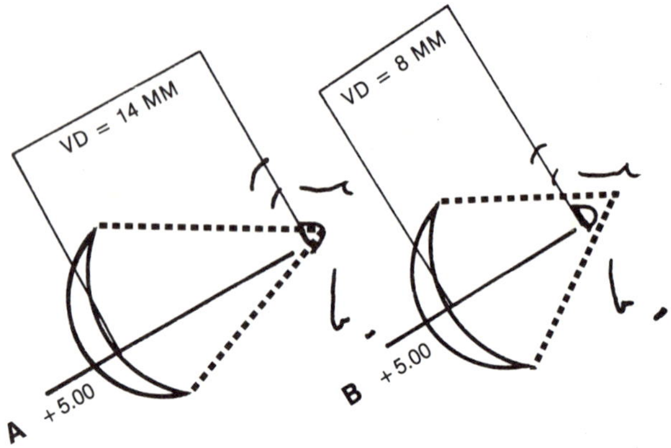

Answer 1252. None required. (This story gets better!)

Frame 1253. *Continued* . . . So they place it in a safe place on the shelf. Several days later the job is sent back to you and you find the P.D. 'somewhat improved'. What happened?

Data: Rx O.D. +1.00 −1.00 × 90
O.S. +2.00 −4.00 × 135
56/18 Rectangular Shape
P.D. 63
Lensometer ink spot P.D. = 68

Question: What is the consequence of failing to decenter for P.D. by 5 mm.? Why the difference in the lab P.D. and yours?

Answer 839. **−1.00.**

Frame 840. There are −1.00 diopters of power at axis 090 in the Rx −2.00 +1.00 × 180. The rules for crossed cylinder form state: Combine the opposite axis with the power in a given meridian. Study the illustration in this frame.

Since the 090 axis was chosen, the power to be combined lies on the opposite axis. This power is **(−1.00/−2.00)**.

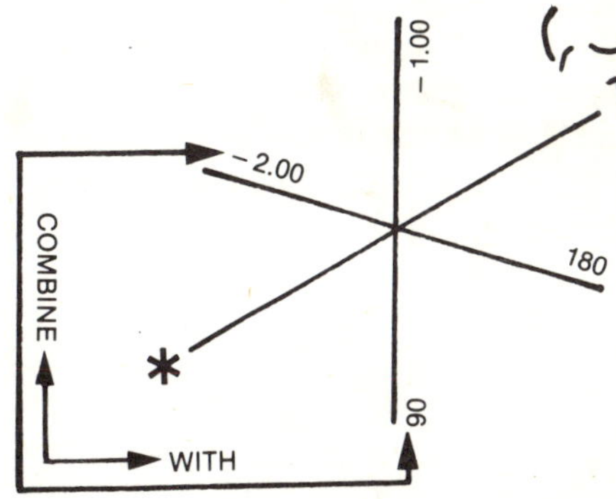

Answer 977. **Is, upward, creating.**

Frame 978. When the eye turns downward to read, the effect is as if the lens was decentered upward and a prismatic effect occurs. Mentally 'look' through this lens once again. This time, 'look' to your left.

As you do the effect is as if the lens was decentered **(out/in)**.

Answer 1115. Behind.

Frame 1116. If the point of focus is to be on the retina, the lens in example B in the last frame will read **(more/less)** plus in order to focus it exactly on the retina.

Answer 1253. Please continue . . .

Frame 1254. Analyzing this Rx at axis 180 reveals:

Calculation: O.D. +1.00 −1.00 × 90
Study the illustration for O.D. in this frame.

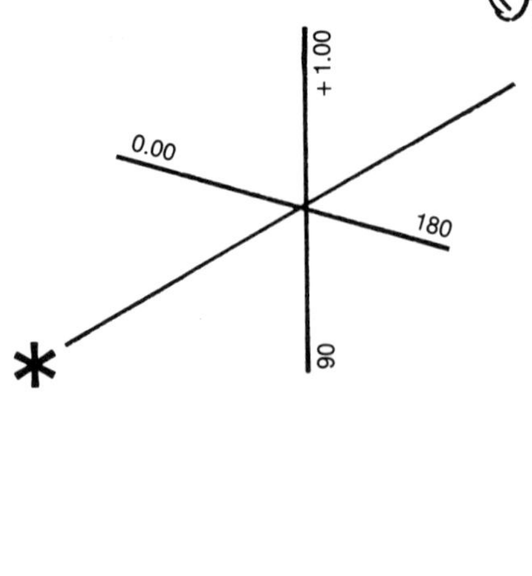

Power in the horizontal meridian is **(0.00/+1.00)** and **(some/no)** decentration is effective. O.S. +2.00 −4.00 × 135 has how much total power at 180? = +2.00 + (50% of −4.00) = 0. Can the Optical center of this Rx be found in the lensometer? **(Yes/No)**

Answer 840. **−2.00.**

Frame 841. The rules for crossed cylinder form say: Combine the *power* in a given axis meridian with the *axis* of the opposite meridian.

The power in the 090 axis meridian of the Rx −2.00 +1.00 × 180 is −1.00, therefore, the opposite axis to be used is not 090, but **(100/180)**.

Answer 978. **In.**

Frame 979. Looking to your left through the left lens creates an effect as if the lens was decentered in. If you are looking 10 mm. to the left, then the prismatic effect of the Rx +2.00 +1.00 × 90 becomes

$$\Delta = \frac{d \times P}{10} = \frac{(10) \times (+3.00)}{10} = 3.00.$$

Plus lenses are considered to be two prisms base to base. Study the illustration in this frame. The dotted line representing the O.S. looking 10 mm. to the left is looking through a Δ whose base is in. The prismatic effect, then, is called **(base in/base out)**.

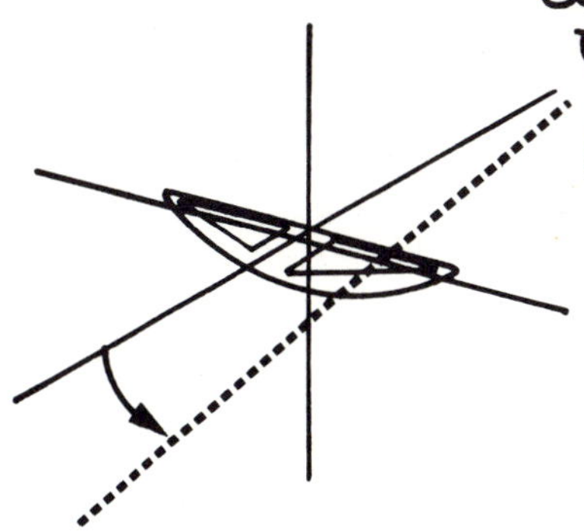

Answer 1116. More.

Frame 1117. Now, think about this. If more plus had to be added, then the effective power of the lens had to have become **(stronger/weaker)** as the vertex distance changed from 14 mm. to 8 mm.

Answer 1254. 0.00, No, No.

Frame 1255. The Rx O.D. +1.00 −1.00 × 90
O.S. +2.00 −4.00 × 135
can be 'spotted' in many different places along the plano horizontal meridian. By simply holding the Rx up and observing 'movement,' the Optician would have known this to be plano at 180.

So, the deadly Rx raises its evil axis once again, this time causing a **(necessary/unnecessary)** delay and questionable effect on the lab/dispenser relationship.

Answer 841. 180. (Stay with it!)

Frame 842. The combination of opposite axis with a given power meridian yields the crossed cylinder form. Study the illustration in this frame.

The opposite combination of −1.00 is axis 180, the opposite combination of −2.00 is **(090/045).**

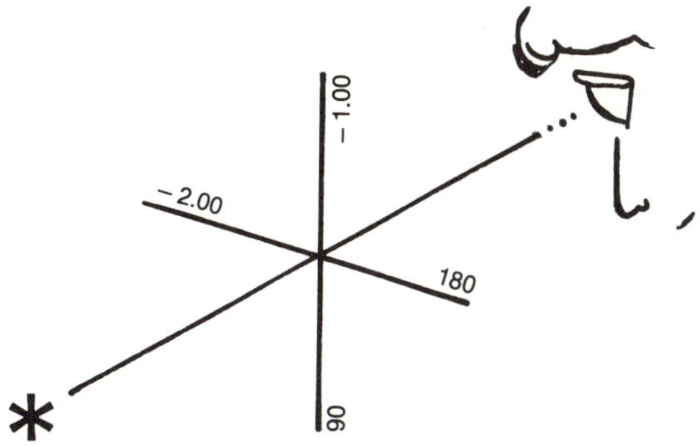

Answer 979. Base in.

Frame 980. Looking 10 mm. to the left through O.S. +2.00 +1.00 × 90 creates a prismatic effect of 3.00 Δ B.I. Looking 8 mm. down creates 1.6 Δ B.U.

Now, mentally 'look' through your lens up *and* outward at axis 135. The power at this point becomes **(+2.50/+2.00/+1.00).**

Answer 1117. Weaker. (Don't just guess! Really think about it.)

Frame 1118. A plus 5.00 became effectively weaker as the vertex distance became less, that is, shorter. Study the example in this frame. It illustrates a −8.00 sph with two different vertex distances. The lens in example B is **(closer/further)** from the eye.

The focus of example B is therefore **(in front of/behind)** the retina.

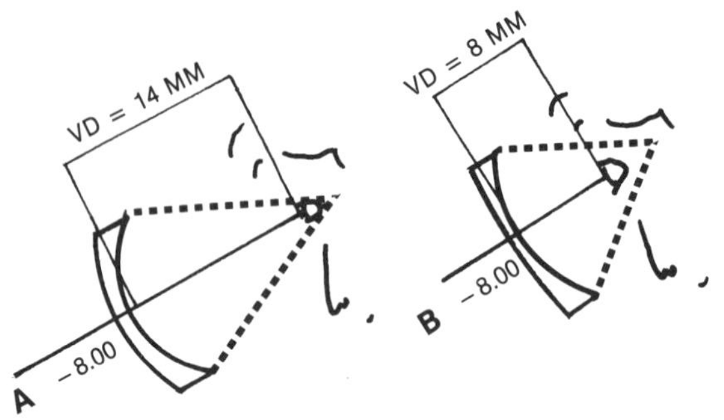

Answer 1255. Unnecessary.

Frame 1256.

Title: **THE DOCTOR'S RE-CHECK**

Situation: Two weeks ago, you dispensed a beautifully and perfectly checked out pair of glasses. Your patient tried to get used to the new Rx but felt uncomfortable. Instead of returning directly to you, the patient returned to the Doctor. The Doctor's assistant verified the prescription and found the P.D. off by 10 mm. and vertical imbalance of 1.00 B.U. The patient now returns to you, bearing a very important note from the Doctor . . . "Dear Optician . . . Fix it!"

Data: Rx O.D. −1.00 +4.00 × 30
O.S. −1.50 +3.00 × 135 P.D. = 64

Question: 1. Can you? **(Yes/No)**
2. Should you? **(Yes/No)**.

Frame 56/14 — Aviator Shape — Lensometer Spots P.D. = 74

Answer 842. 090. Crossed cylinders are easy as pie!

Frame 843. The crossed cylinder form of −2.00 +1.00 × 180 is written −1.00 × 180 ⊙ −2.00 × 090. Opticians read this, "minus one at one-eighty combined with a minus two at ninety." The crossed cylinder expression may also be read as "minus two at ninety combined with minus one at one-eighty."

There are **(one/two)** correct ways of expressing crossed cylinder notation.

Answer 980. +2.50.

Frame 981. The Optician can analyze sphero-cylindrical lenses to predict the optical effects as the eyes travel from one point to another. Through careful observation and discussion of exactly how the lenses will be used, the dispensing Optician can better help the patient to understand his/her own prescription. Now, consider two lenses: The Rx

O.D. −2.00 +3.00 × 90
O. S. −2.00 +3.00 × 180

Continue to mentally picture this Rx in front of your own eyes. Power horizontally and vertically for this Rx is **(equal/unequal)**.

Answer 118. Closer, behind.

Frame 1119. Since the lens focus in example B is behind the retina, plus must be added to bring the focus back onto the retina. From the examples in Frame 1113-1119, the Optician can see that, in order to compensate for a plus lens vertex becoming shorter, plus must also be added. The Optician can also see that for a minus lens vertex distance becoming less plus must also be added.

Thus, it can be concluded that anytime a lens is moved closer to the eye (vertex shortened), plus must be **(added/subtracted)** in order to compensate.

____

Answer 1256. Yes, No. (How come?)

Frame 1257.

Solution: Horizontal meridian analysis

O.D. −1.00 +4.00 × 30 = ? × 180

(−1.00) + (25% +4.00) at 180

(−1.00) + (+1.00) = 0.00 × 180

O.S. −1.50 +3.00 × 135

(−1.50) + (50% +3.00) at 180

(−1.50) + (+1.50) = 0.00 × 180

Measuring the incorrect P.D. by trying to use the lensometer is **(easy/difficult)** to do.

Question: Why is there vertical imbalance?

____

Answer 843. Two.

Frame 844. The crossed cylinders $-1.00 \times 180 \odot -2.00 \times 090$ are two cylinder Rx's which, when combined, form the Rx illustrated in this frame. The Optician can mentally visualize the crossed cylinder form on a visual line of sight in the same manner as a conventional Rx.

Crossed cylinders are mentally visualized the same as plus or **(minus/mindless)** cylinder Rx's.

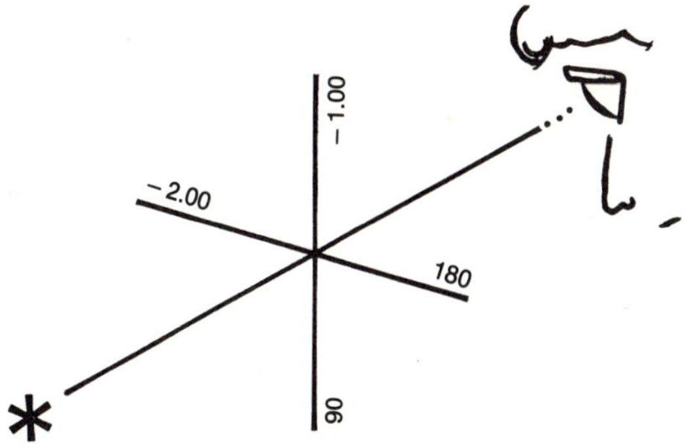

Answer 981. Unequal.

Frame 982. *Please continue* . . . As your eyes look 10 mm. to the right, a combined effect takes place.

$$\text{O.D. } \Delta = \frac{d \times P}{10} = \frac{(10)\times(+1.00)}{10} = 1.00 \text{ B.I. and}$$

$$\text{O.S. } \Delta = \frac{d \times P}{10} = \frac{(10)\times(-2.00)}{10} = 2.00 \text{ B.O.}$$

O.D. +O.S. = 3 Δ B.I.

Suppose you looked down at a point 8 mm. below the O.C. to read.

The effect O.D. will be

$$\Delta = \frac{d \times P}{10} = \frac{(8)\times(-2.00)}{10} = 1.6 \text{ B.D.}$$

The effect O.S. will be

$$\Delta = \frac{d \times P}{10} = \frac{(8)\times(+1.00)}{10} = .8 \text{ B.U.}$$

The **(single/combined)** optical prismatic effect, then, will be 1.6 + 0.8 = 2.4.

Answer 1119. Added.

Frame 1120. Just exactly how much plus must be added for vertex distance compensation can be calculated utilizing the focal length and Dioptric power formulas:

$$f = \frac{1000}{D} \text{ and } D = \frac{1000}{f}.$$

If an original prescription +9.50 was at 14 mm. vertex distance and, due to frame change, the lens wound up at 9 mm. vertex distance, what plus power will compensate for the difference?

To answer the question, the Optician must first calculate the focal length of +9.50, $f = \frac{1000}{D}$

$$f = \frac{1000}{+9.50}$$

$$f = 105 \text{ mm.}$$

Secondly, the Optician now needs a lens whose focal length will be the difference between the original vertex and the changed vertex. That number is **(5/22)**.

Answer 1257. Easy.

Frame 1258. *Comment:* As seen in Chapter 13, when oblique axis lenses are decentered horizontally, the optical centers drift apart vertically. Reading the lenses in the lensometer, the assistant arbitrarily happened to select a point far enough out on the horizontal meridian to induce an apparent imbalance. If the P.D. were first 'dotted' with the glasses on the patient's face, and then set in the lensometer, then evil Mr. Prism would not have appeared and **(some/no)** vertical imbalance would show and the P.D. would be **(correct/still off)**.

Answer 844. Minus.

Frame 845. Study the illustration in this frame. The illustration shows the combining of two crossed cylinders.

The third cross represents the sum of the combination of the two crossed **(cylinders/spheres)**.

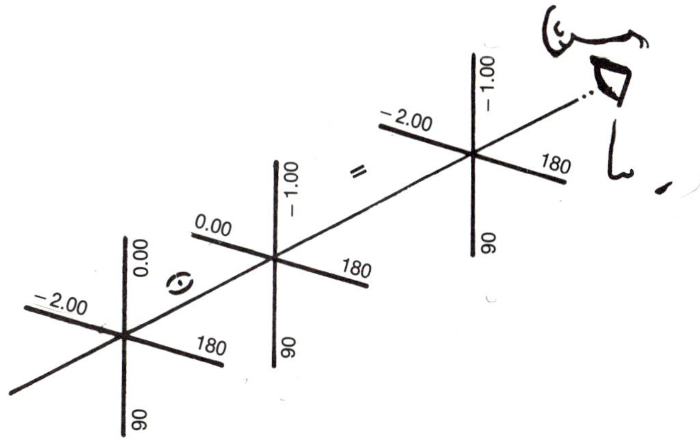

$-2.00 \times 90 \odot -1.00 \times 180$

Answer 982. Combined.

Frame 983. The brain combines the two focused images (O.D. & O.S.) into a single picture.

When there is a significant difference between these two individual images, the brain **(may have/ never has)** difficulty.

Answer 1120. 5.

Frame 1121. The changed vertex distance is 5 mm. less than the original 14 mm. A +9.50 has a focal length of 105 mm. But, the lens power now needed will have to have a focus 100 mm.

Therefore . . . 105 − 5 = 100 mm.

What is the Dioptric Power of a lens whose focal length is 100 mm.? Would you use formula **(A/B)**?

A) $D = \frac{1000}{f}$ B) $f = \frac{1000}{D}$

Answer 1258. No, correct.

Frame 1259. Do you think that a conversation with the Doctor where you could explain the problem, along with the solution, might save re-making glasses and causing the patient to doubt your indispensable skills? **(Yes/No)** Do you think the Doctor will be impressed with your optical knowledge and consult you on other problems? **(Yes/No)** Do you think the Doctor might be receptive to your teaching the art of lensometry to the office assistants, thus saving time and possible patient dissatisfaction? **(Yes/No)**

Answer 845. Cylinders.

Frame 846. The result of combining two crossed cylinders can be a compound prescription or a simple spherical prescription. Study the example in this frame. The example asks you to combine the two cylinders −3.00 × 90 with −3.00 × 180.

The result will be a **(sphere/cylinder)** Rx.

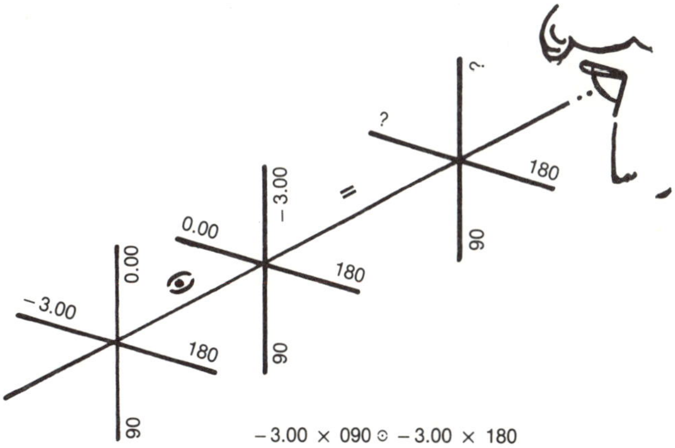

Answer 983. May have.

Frame 984. The brain may have difficulty in bringing two images together when they are very different. As a general rule, when there is a horizontal difference of 1.00 △ or a vertical difference of 0.50 △, problems may occur.

This rule is **(specified/general)** and will **(differ/remain the same)** for each individual.

Answer 1121. A.

Frame 1122. $D = \frac{1000}{F} = \frac{1000}{100} = +10.00.$

The Dioptric power of a lens whose focal length is 100 mm. is +10.00 D. Turn the page to Frame 1123.

Answer 1259. Yes, Yes, Yes. (What do you mean, I don't know your doctor?)

Frame 1260.

Title: **PERPLEXING PRISM**

Situation: A lovable, frail golden-ager settles into the chair at your dispensing table. With a twinkle in her eye, she asks that you duplicate her present glasses with a more contemporary frame style. She thinks she has 'prism glasses' and has been told to be very careful of whomever makes glasses for her. Since you work in a state that prohibits duplication without a prescription, and her last examination was more than three years ago, you arrange for another examination. The Doctor instructs you to . . .

Answer 846. sphere

Frame 847. A −3.00 × 090 ⊙ −3.00 × 180 results in a −3.00 sphere. Demonstrate your knowledge of crossed cylinder form by correctly matching the Rx on the right with the crossed cylinder form on the left.

A) −3.50 × 180 ⊙ −1.00 × 090	1) −2.00 sph
B) −2.00 × 090 ⊙ −2.00 × 180	2) −3.50 +2.50 × 090
C) +1.75 × 045 ⊙ −2.75 × 135	3) +1.75 −4.50 × 135
D) +1.00 × 160 ⊙ +4.00 × 070	4) +1.00 +3.00 × 070

Answer 984. General, Differ

Frame 985. Although tolerance of 1.00 Δ of induced prismatic effect horizontally and 0.50 Δ of induced prismatic effect vertically may differ with each individual, Opticians use it as a guide to predict or substantiate problems with the lenses.

As long as the combined prismatic effect remains within the guidelines, there will seldom be problems. Once the combined effect exceeds those guidelines, the dispenser **(should/shouldn't)** be wary.

Answer 1122. You are doing fine; stay with it!

Frame 1123. Opticians use the abbreviation V.D. for vertex distance. V.D. = 14, means Vertex Distance 14 millimeters. When compensatig for V.D. in simple prescriptions, the Optician first calculates the focal length in millimeters. Secondly, the difference between the two V.D.'s is found and the result is either added or subtracted (depending upon whether the needed lens is closer or further from the eye) from the original focal length. Thirdly, the needed focal length is re-converted into diopters and fourthly, the answer is rounded off to the nearest practical Diopter.

The preceeding description consists of **(floor/four)** steps.

Answer 1260. Please Continue . . .

Frame 1261. "Duplicate exact prism as patient is wearing."

Data: Rx O.D. −0.75 +1.00 × 120
O.S. Plano +2.75 × 180
ADD +2.00

Frame 53/16 Upsweep Shape
P.D. 58/55

Question:

1. Can lensometry alone reveal vertical prism? **(Yes/No)**
2. Can lensometry alone reveal horizontal prism? **(Yes/No)**

Solution 1:
O.D. −0.75 + (25% of +1.00) = −0.50 at 90
O.S. Plano + (100% of +2.75) = +2.75 at 90

Answer 847. A 2, B 1, C 3, D 4.

Frame 848. Continue your self test by correctly completing the chart below. The chart shows an Rx in the lensometer and asks you to read the required form.

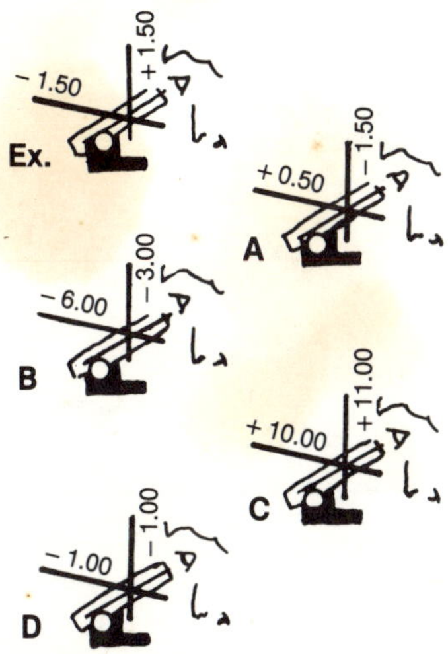

MINUS CYL	PLUS CYL	CROSSED CYLINDER
Ex. +1.50 −3.00 × 90	−1.50 +3.00 × 180	−1.50 × 90 ⊙ +1.50 × 180 OR +1.50 × 180 ⊙ −1.50 × 90
A		
B		
C		
D		

Answer 985. Should.

Frame 986. Study the Rx in this frame.

O.D. +2.00 Sphere
O.S. +4.00 Sphere

As the line of sight passes directly through the Optical Centers of this Rx, the prismatic effect is **(Δ 2.00/Δ 0.00)**. As they look upward 8 mm., as might be required for a certain job, the combined prismatic effect is:

$$\text{O.D. } \Delta = \frac{d \times P}{10} = \frac{(8) \times (+2.00)}{10} = 1.6 \text{ B.D.}$$

and

$$\text{O.S. } \Delta = \frac{d \times P}{10} = \frac{(8) \times (+4.00)}{10} = 3.2 \text{ B.D.}$$

The net prismatic effect will be the *difference* between 3.2 and 1.6 or **(1.6/4.8)**.

Answer 1123. Four. (I know that seems like a lot of steps.)

Frame 1124. Test your skill at calculating the required lens power for the vertex distance problems in this frame. Compare your answers with the correct ones in Frame 1125.

Rx	f = 1000/D	PREVIOUS VD − NEW VD = DIFFERENCE	f ± DIFFERENCE = NEEDED f (In MM)	D = 1000/f = EXACT D	PRACTICAL D
Ex: +8.00	f =125 mm.	15 mm. − 10 mm. = 5 mm.	125 − 5 = 120	$D = \frac{1000}{120}$ = 8.33	+8.37
A) +10.50	?	14 mm. − 11 mm. = 3 mm.	? = ?	? = ?	?
B) −11.00	?	13 mm. − 9 mm. = 4 mm.	? = ?	? = ?	?
C) −12.50	?	11 mm. − 14 mm. = 3 mm.	? = ?	? = ?	?
D) +14.00	?	10 mm. − 12 mm. = 2 mm.	? = ?	? = ?	?

Answer 1261. Yes, No. (Not in this Rx.) Please Continue.

Frame 1262. The Rx for analysis purpose now becomes:

O.D. −0.50 in the 90° meridian
O.S. +2.75 in the 90° meridian

The rule for Rx verification is: Check out the stronger lens first. If no vertical imbalance shows, then no vertical imbalance exists! If you check the O.S. first, will there be imbalance? **(Yes/No)**. Now, for the horizontal meridian.

2. O.D. −0.75 +1.00 × 120 = ? × 180
   O.S. Plano +2.75 × 180 = ? × 180

   O.D. −0.75 + (75% of +1.00) = 0.00 × 180
   O.S. Plano + (0% of +2.75) = 0.00 × 180

If prism exists at 180, then it **(could/could not)** have been achieved thru decentration.

Answer 848. Answers to Frame 848 below.

Frame 849.

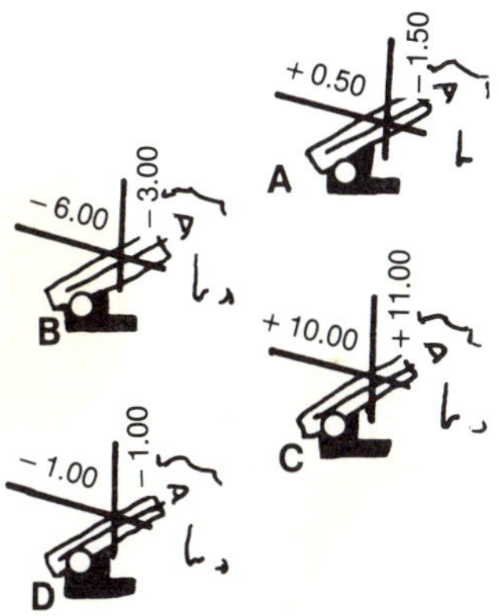

	MINUS CYL	PLUS CYL	CROSSED CYLINDER
A	+0.50 −2.00 × 180	−1.50 +2.00 × 90	−1.50 × 180 ⊙ +0.50 × 90 OR +0.50 × 90 ⊙ −1.50 × 180
B	−3.00 −3.00 × 90	−6.00 +3.00 × 180	−6.00 × 90 ⊙ −3.00 × 180 OR −3.00 × 180 ⊙ −6.00 × 90
C	+11.00 −1.00 × 90	+10.00 +1.00 × 180	+10.00 × 90 ⊙ +11.00 × 180 OR +11.00 × 180 ⊙ +10.00 × 90
D	N/A	N/A	−1.00 × 90 ⊙ −1.00 × 180 OR −1.00 × 180 ⊙ −1.00 × 90

Answer 986. **△ 0.00, 1.6.**

Frame 987. *Differences* in the prismatic effect of vertical meridians are called vertical imbalances. The Optician can compensate (re-balance) the vertical imbalance by adjusting the **(vertical/horizontal)** position of the optical centers.

Consider the Rx O.D. +3.00 −2.00 × 180
O.S. +4.00 −1.50 × 90

If the eyes were lowered to read at a point of 8 mm. below the optical centers, the total vertical imbalance would be **(4.2/2.4)** base **(down/up)**.

Answer 1124. Are below in Frame 1125. How did you do?

. . . .

Frame 1125.

Rx	$f = \frac{1000}{D}$	PREVIOUS VD – NEW VD = DIFFERENCE	f ± DIFFERENCE = NEEDED f (In MM)	$D = \frac{1000}{f}$ = EXACT D	PRACTICAL D
Ex: +8.00	f =125 mm.	15 mm. − 10 mm. = 5 mm.	125 − 5 = 120.0 mm.	$D = \frac{1000}{120.0} = 8.33$	+8.37
A) +10.50	f = 95.2	14 mm. − 11 mm. = 3 mm.	95.2 − 3 = 92.2	$D = \frac{1000}{92.2} = 10.84$	+10.87
B) −11.00	f = 90.9	13 mm. − 9 mm. = 4 mm.	90.9 + 4 = 94.9	$D = \frac{1000}{94.9} = 10.53$	−10.50
C) −12.50	f = 80.0	11 mm. − 14 mm. = 3 mm.	80.0 − 3 = 77.0	$D = \frac{1000}{77.0} = 12.98$	−13.00
D) +14.00	f = 71.4	10 mm. − 12 mm. = 2 mm.	71.4 + 2 = 73.4	$D = \frac{1000}{73.4} = 13.62$	+13.62

Answer 1262. No, Could Not.

. . . .

Frame 1263. *Comment:* If prism could not have been achieved thru decentration, then it must be ground in prism. Returning to the problem . . . Ascertaining horizontal prism can be accomplished by spotting the P.D.'s with a felt-tip pen as the patient looks through the glasses. Placing the marked dot in the lensometer at the geometric center of the aperture will insure a proper reading. If prism shows as the centered lens is read, the prism indeed **(exists/persists)**. The Optician can satisfy both doctor and patient by ascertaining and duplicating the previous prism.

Answer 849. No answer needed. Go to Frame 850.

Frame 850. In lower power lenses crossed or conventional cylinder form is considered equivalent. In higher prescriptions, especially strong cylinders, crossed cylinder form may provide not only the best-looking lens, but the *only* way the prescription may be made.

By splitting the cylinder on both sides of the lens, the Optician can design a cosmetically acceptable and optically functional **(lens/len)**.

Answer 987. Vertical, 2.4, up.

Frame 988. Analyze your answer:

$$\text{O.D. } \Delta = \frac{d \times P}{10} = \frac{(8) \times (+1.00)}{10} = 0.8 \text{ B.U.}$$

$$\text{O.S. } \Delta = \frac{d \times P}{10} = \frac{(8) \times (+4.00)}{10} = 3.2 \text{ B.U.}$$

Therefore, 3.2 − 0.8 = 2.4 B.U.

Since the **(O.D./O.S.)** is stronger, the effect becomes 2.4 B.U. more prismatic effect in that eye than the other eye. If you were to compensate for this, the logical approach would seem to be to 'balance' the 2.4 Δ B.U. with **(2.4^{Δ} B.I./2.4^{Δ} B.D.)**

Answer 1125. None required. Go to next frame.

Frame 1126. With simple Rx's the computations are straight forward, as illustrated in the last several frames. When compound lenses are used, however, the calculation must be separate for each meridian. Study the example in this frame.

O.D. +15.00 +1.00 × 90 VD = 13

If the patient chooses a frame with a VD = 10 mm., what power must be ordered from the lab? The Optician begins by choosing the sphere meridian first. The power of the sphere is **(+16.00/ +15.00)**. Secondly, the cylinder meridian is calculated and the new Rx is plotted on a visual line of sight graph.

Answer 1263. Exists.

Frame 1264.

Title: **ANISOMETROPIC ANOMOLIES**

Situation: You are having a very good day. It has been one of those fabulous afternoons where just everyone seems to appreciate you (even your boss!). This particular afternoon you are writing up orders to send to the lab. Even though you did not dispense this Rx, something stops you and you focus on the data.

Data: Rx O.D. +3.00 +2.00 × 180
O.S. +2.00 +1.75 × 90
ADD +2.50

Answer 850. Lens.

Frame 851.

CHAPTER 6
BASE CURVES SELECTION

TURN TO THE TOP OF PAGE 191, **FRAME 852**

Answer 988. O.S., 2.4$^{\Delta}$B.D.

Frame 989. 2.4$^{\Delta}$B.D. will balance out 2.4 B.U. Therefore, the objective with vertical imbalance is to determine decentration necessary to achieve this. The formula to find decentration is $d = \frac{10\,\Delta}{P}$. Refer to the Rx in Frame 987 once again. Which vertical power would you use? **(A/B).**

A) $d = \frac{10 \times \Delta}{P} = \frac{10 \times 2.4}{+1.00}$

B) $d = \frac{10 \times \Delta}{P} = \frac{10 \times 2.4}{+4.00}$

Answer 1126. +15.00.

Frame 1127. A +15.00 has a focal length of $f = \frac{1000}{15.00} = 66.6$ mm. Study the steps in this frame.

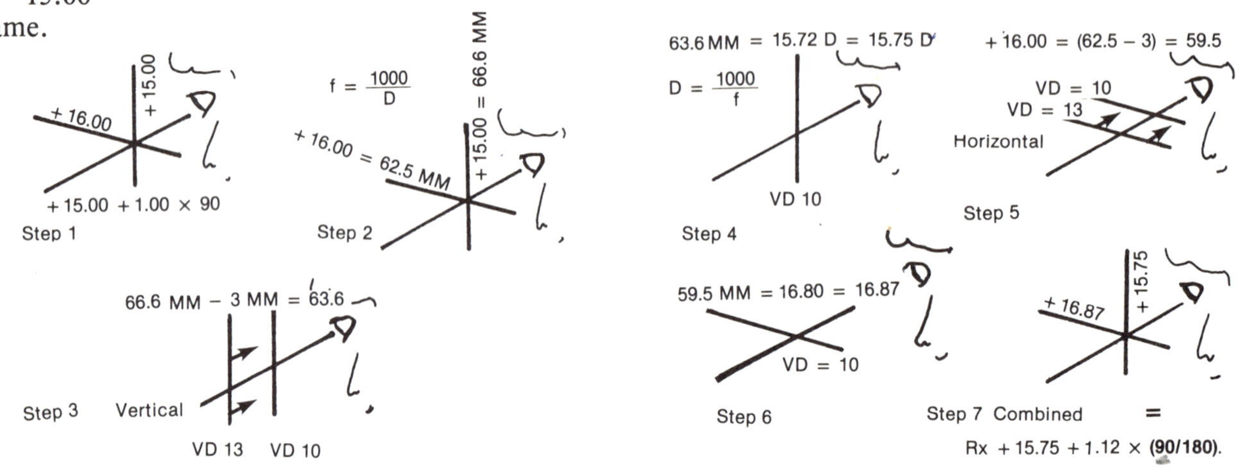

Answer 1264. None required.

Frame 1265. As you begin to fill out the paperwork, you realize that this Rx is deceptive; on the surface it seems innocuous. If it hadn't been for the fact that you had just finished reading *OPTICIANRY: The Practice and the Art, Vol. II — The Science*, you might have passed it over as an everyday garden variety Rx, but there was something curious about the powers, so you began to analyze.

Question: 1. Could there be any problem with the Horizontal Meridian? **(Yes/No)**

2. Could there be any problem with the Vertical Meridian? **(Yes/No)**

Answer 851. None required.

Frame 852. Recommended base curve choice for any given lens power will vary slightly from manufacturers to manufacturers, each with their own scientific proof with complex formulae. The dispensing Optician who relies upon his supplier for base curve guidance is usually guided correctly because the lab has the manufacturers' recommended base curve charts.

The lab uses recommended base curve **(carts/charts).**

Answer 989. B.

Frame 990. The vertical lens power of +4.00 is strongest and will need to have the optical center moved so as to create 2.4 △ B.D. Follow the mathematics:

$$d = \frac{10 \times \Delta}{P} = \frac{(10) \times (2.4)}{+4.00} = \frac{24}{4} = 6 \text{ mm.}$$

By **(lowering/raising)** the O.S. O.C. 6 mm., the vertical imbalance created at a point 8 mm. below the optical centers of the Rx:

O.D. +3.00 −2.00 × 180
O.S. +4.00 −1.50 × 90

will be re-balanced.

Answer 1127. 90.

Frame 1128. The Rx +15.00 +1.00 × 90 VD = 14 must be compensated with plus as it moves 3 mm. closer to the eye. The Optician first calculates each meridian separately, then combines the results and 'reads' the lens needed for compensation. See if you can remember the steps without looking back.

1. The Optician first converts Diopters to **(millimeters/centimeters)** in each meridian.

2. The difference between previous V.D. and **(new/old)** V.D. is calculated.

3. The decision as to what millimeter focus is **(never/now)** needed is determined.

4. Millimeters are converted back to Diopters using the formula $\mathbf{(D = \frac{1000}{f} / \frac{1000}{D})}$.

5. The **(compensated/complicated)** Rx is ordered.

Answer 1265. No, yes.

Frame 1266. *Solution:* The prismatic effect of an average reading level 8 mm. below the distance O.D. will produce:

O.D. +3.00 + (100%of +2.00) = +5.00 at 90

$$\Delta = \frac{d \times P}{10}$$

$$\Delta = \frac{+5.00 \times 8}{10} = \frac{40}{10} = 4.0\ \Delta \text{ Base Up}$$

O.S. +2.00 + (0% of +1.75) = +2.00 at 90

$$\Delta = \frac{d \times P}{10}$$

$$\Delta = \frac{+2.00 \times 8}{10} = \frac{16}{10} = 1.6\ \Delta \text{ Base Up}$$

The net prismatic effect is **(5.6 B.U./2.4 B.U.) (O.D./O.S.)**.

Answer 852. Charts.

Frame 853. In the absence of base curve guidelines, that is, a previous known curve or a chart, the Optician may use a rule of thumb formula. Study the diagram in the next frame (number 854). The diagram illustrates Vogel's formula for basic base curve selection.

The base curve selector chart represents **(Vogel's/ Bird's)** formula.

Answer 990. Lowering.

Frame 991. A vertical imbalance created (induced) at a given point of a pair of glasses requires balancing only if the eyes were to remain in that position for a period of time. As long as the visual axis remains near, or close enough to the optical centers so as not to induce Δ 1.00 horizontal or Δ 0.50 vertical imbalances, all will be well. Study the illustration in this frame.

The illustration shows two ways an object may be viewed. One by lowering the eyes (A) and the other by lowering the **(head/feet)** (B).

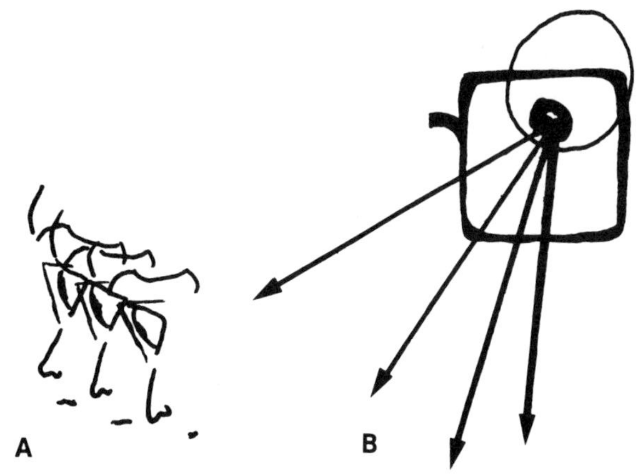

Answer 1128. Millimeters, new, now, $D = \frac{1000}{f}$, compensated.

Frame 1129. Vertex distance compensation has many applications in Opticianry. The precise focal length and dioptric power formulas are used to order the exact lens needed. The lab has special charts which calculate the entire diopter and Vertex Distance range. The Optician can use an 'approximate' Vertex Distance formula, though, for quick calculation at the dispensing table.

This formula arrives at the amount of Dioptric change related to millimeters of change. Here is the formula: $D_c = \frac{mmm.}{1000} \times D^2$.

This formula is **(precise/approximate).**

____

Answer 1266. 2.4 B.U., O.D.

Frame 1267. There is 2.4 △ B.U. O.D., which is enough vertical imbalance to cause problems. Since you did not take in the job, however, you begin to explore with the following questions:

1. What was the past Rx?
2. Was the past Rx compensated?
3. Does the patient have usable vision in the other eye?
4. Does the doctor wish this to be compensated?

The answers to your questions were:

1. None 2. No 3. Yes 4. Please

You can compensate with one of **(two/five)** methods.

____

Answer 853. Vogel's.

Frame 854. Vogel's formula works on spherical equivalent.

Turn to Frame 855.

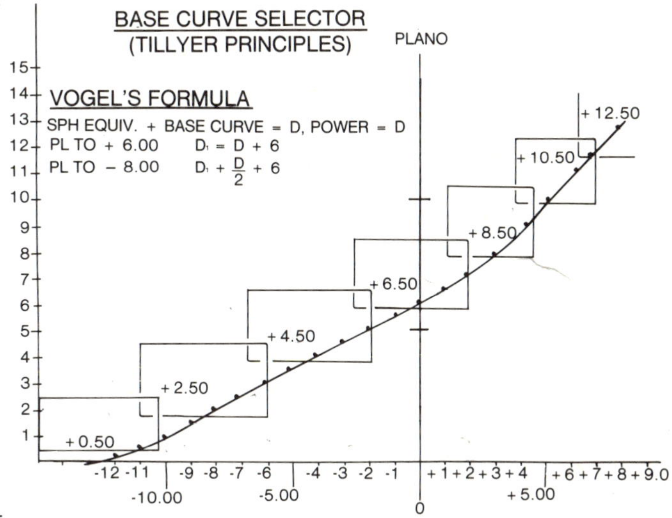

Answer 991. Head.

Frame 992. If the head is lowered, then the eyes remain fixed through the optical centers and **(no/some)** imbalance occurs. If, on the other hand, the eyes themselves are lowered, then the induced prismatic vertical imbalance will appear and the O.C. of the lenses **(need/don't need)** compensation.

Answer 1129. Approximate.

Frame 1130. The 'approximate' vertex distance formula is $D_c = \frac{\text{mmm.}}{1000} \times P^2$.

where: D_c = Diopter change
mmm. = Millimeters moved
P^2 = Power squared (Power times Power)

Here is how it works: A +13.50 sph is moved 3 mm. further from the eye.

$$D_c = \frac{\text{mmm.}}{1000} \times P^2$$

$$D_c = \frac{3}{1000} \times 13.50^2$$

$$D_c = \frac{3}{1000} \times 182.25$$

D_c = 54.6 or a fraction over 0.50 D

The amount of change is about 0.50. Do you think this lens has become 0.50 D **(stronger/weaker)**?

Answer 1267. Five.

Frame 1268. There are five methods of compensating for vertical imbalance. The correct one will be the one which is in the best interests of the patient from a financial, cosmetic and optical standpoint. After careful discussion with the patient, you decide to slab off the **(O.D./O.S.)** with base up prism. Because you know that it is always best to prescribe less than the total needed, you instruct the lab to grind slab off **(1.00/2.00)**.

Answer 854. No answer required.

Frame 855. Vogel's formula combines the best of many charts and uses the spherical equivalent as a basis.

Vogel's chart uses the **(spiritual/spherical)** equivalent.

Answer 992. No, need.

Frame 993. Think back to the Rx in Frame 987. If the patient had a visual need to view objects at a point below the optical centers for a prolonged period of time AND that person could not conveniently lower their head, you would best serve that patient by **(compensating/forgetting)** the Rx.

Answer 1130. Stronger.

Frame 1131. A +13.50 becomes (one-half diopter) 0.50 stronger as it is moved 3 mm. further from the eye. Try another one: A −10.50 is moved 3 mm. closer to the eye.

$$D_c = \frac{\text{mmm.}}{1000} \times P_2$$

$$D_c = \frac{4}{1000} \times 10.50$$

$$D_c = .004 \times 10.50$$

$$D_c = 0.44 \quad \text{or } .50$$

Is this new effective power **(−11.00/−10.00)**.

Answer 1268. O.S., 2.00.

Frame 1269. *Comment:* Without careful prescription analysis, this Rx might not have been noticed. The patient may have never returned, thinking that 'your' glasses didn't work well and always caused discomfort. Oftentimes when patients complain of asthenopia, they really do have something the matter.

Failure to explore beyond routine verification **(cannot/can)** lead to an unhappy **(Optician/patient)**.

Answer 855. Spherical.

Frame 856. The spherical equivalent is calculated by adding one-half of the cylinder power to the sphere power. Study the example in this frame. The example shows the Rx −2.00 +1.00 × 180. One-half the +1.00 cylinder is +0.50. A −2.00 added to a +0.50 = −1.50.

Ex. −2.00 +1.00 × 180 = −1.50 spherical equivalent

Adding the sphere power to one-half the cylinder power yields the spherical **(equal/equivalent)**.

Answer 993. Compensating.

Frame 994. Look back at the Rx in Frame 987 once again. Which case below would you consider to be a problem due to vertical imbalance? **(A/B)**?

A) Case History: Patient works on an assembly line and is seated. The job requires inserting a wire in a slot and placing it in a bin while monitoring an electric light which is above eye level.

B) Case History: Patient works at eye level, pushing buttons on a switchboard mounted chest high.

Answer 1131. **−11.00.**

Frame 1132. If the effective power of −10.50 moved 3 mm. closer to the eye becomes −11.00, then the Optician compensates by **(adding/subtracting)** +0.50 and orders **(−10.00/−11.50)**.

Answer 1269. **Can, either or both Optician and patient.**

Frame 1270.

Title: **TWO DIFFERENT EYES IN THE SAME HEAD**

Situation: You have known this 70-year-old gentleman for many years. You have helped counsel him when you 'knew' he was getting cataracts, as well as pre- and post-operatively, when his patience was low and he kept asking you if you knew when the doctor was going to prescribe glasses.

Now the day has come. You study the Rx and data.

Answer 856. Equivalent.

Frame 857. The spherical equivalent of −2.00 +1.00 × 180 is −1.50. Test your skill at calculating spherical equivalents by correctly completing the chart below.

	Rx		Spherical Equivalent
Ex:	+3.00 −2.00 × 90	=	+2.00
A)	−4.50 +0.50 × 180	=	?
B)	+1.50 +4.00 × 165	=	?
C)	−0.25 +0.50 × 72	=	?
D)	−4.25 −4.00 × 30	=	?

Answer 994. A.

Frame 995. When oblique axis are involved, calculating the prismatic effects, both vertical and horizontal, becomes a bit more complicated because prism is created both up and in or down and out with decentration. At first glance, the Rx:

O.D. −1.00 +4.00 × 30
O.S. −2.00 +4.00 × 45

has a horizontal decentration value of zero. However, not decentering this meridian will create vertical imbalance!

Oblique axis decentration is **(different/the same)** as right angle decentration.

Answer 1132. Adding, – 10.00.

Frame 1133. You can use your knowledge of vertex distance compensation to solve the problem in this frame. A patient wears +12.75 VD = 13 mm. If the patient desires contact lenses, what power should be ordered? (You can do it!)

The vertex distance formula $D_c = \frac{\text{mmm.}}{1000} \times P^2$.

$$D_c = \frac{13}{1000} \times 12.75^2$$

$$D_c = \frac{13}{1000} \times 162.5$$

$$D_c = 0.013 - 162.5$$

$$D_c = 2.11 \text{ or } 2.00$$

The contact lens power to be ordered, then, is **(2.00 + 12.75 = 14.75/2.00 −12.75 = 10.75).**

Answer 1270. Continue . . .

Frame 1271.

Data:

Rx	Base Curve	Thickness	Vertex	Index
O.D. +2.50 sph. over IOL*	+8.25	3.2 mm.	13 mm.	1.523
O.S. +1.00 sph.	+6.50	2.5 mm.	13 mm.	1.523

ADD +2.75
Reading Level 10 mm. below distance O.C.

*intraocular lens

Question: 1. Can you compensate for the Vertical imbalance? **(Yes/No)**

2. Can you compensate for the aniseikonia? **(Yes/No)**

Solution: 1. Slab Off 1.5 O.S.
2. Calculate magnification for each eye.

Answer 857. **A) −4.25** **B) +3.50** **C) Plano** **D) −6.25.**

Frame 858. Study the Base Curve Selector chart in Frame 854 once again. The chart uses the spherical equivalent as a basis. For all plus lenses the formula is: Base Curve = Spherical equivalent plus (+6.00). Now, consider the Rx +3.00 +1.00 × 180. The spherical equivalent is +3.50 which is then added to +6.00. A +3.50 plus (+6.00) = +9.50 Base Curve.

The base curve for the Rx +3.00 +1.00 × 180, then, would be **(+9.50/−9.50)**.

Answer 995. **Different.**

Frame 996. The precise calculations for the combined effect of decentering lenses at oblique axis involves higher mathematics and will be presented in another work. However, the Optician can be guided to the consequences of oblique axis decentration in chart form.

The consequences can be best understood **(without/with)** the use of a chart.

Answer 1133. +14.75.

Frame 1134. When prescriptions are compounded, the Optician still can use the formula $D_c = \frac{\text{mmm.}}{1000} \times P^2$, but in each meridian. Study the problem in this frame.

Data: Rx +12.25 +3.00 × 180 V.D. 12 mm.
Lens worn at 8 mm.

Calculation: $D_c = \frac{\text{mmm.}}{1000} \times P^2$

Vertical:

$$D_c = \frac{4}{1000} \times 15.25^2$$

$$D_c = .004 \times 232.5 = 0.93 \text{ or } 1.00$$

Horizontal:

$$D_c = \frac{4}{1000} \times 12.25^2$$

$$D_c = .004 \times 150.06 = 0.60 = 0.62$$

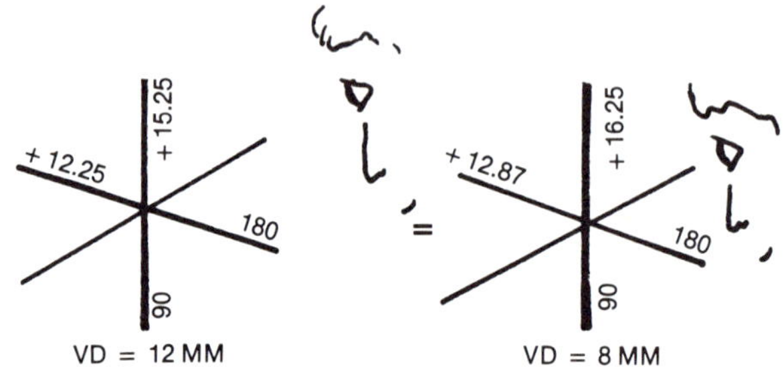

*The Rx in plus cylinder form is ______________

Answer 1271. Yes, yes. Continue . . .

Frame 1272. The formula for magnification:

$$M_t = M_s \times M_p$$

$$M_s = \frac{1}{1 - \frac{(t \times D)}{n}} \qquad M_p = \frac{1}{1 - (dv \times h)}$$

Where

M_t = Total Magnification

M_s = Shape Factor Magnification (base curve, thickness, and index of refraction)

M_p = Power Factor Magnification (vertical distance & power)

t = Thickness (in meters)

n = Index of Refraction

h = Vertex Distance (in meters)

D = Base Curve

D_v = Power

Answer 858. **+9.50.**

Frame 859. For all plus lenses the base curve guide is found by adding +6.00 to the spherical equivalent of the Rx. For all minus lenses: First, divide the spherical equivalent by 2, then add +6.00. Study the example in this frame. The example shows a −4.00 −1.00 × 162 with a spherical equivalent of −4.50, dividing by two and then adding six equals **(+3.75/+6.00).**

−4.00 −1.00 × 162 = −4.50 sph. equiv.

Answer 996. **With.**

Frame 997. Study the two charts in the next two frames. The charts explain the resulting prism when oblique axis Rx's are decentered horizontally and vertically.

HORIZONTAL DECENTRATION (+CYL)

	WHEN	DECENTRATION IN	DECENTRATION OUT
A)	O.D. axis is between 90 and 180 O.S. axis is between 0 and 90	Induces Δ Base Up	Induces Δ Base Down
	O.D. axis is between 0 and 90 O.S. axis is between 90 and 180	Induces Δ Base Down	Induces Δ Base Up

Answer 1134. +12.87 +3.37 × 180.

Frame 1135. Test your skill at Vertex Distance compensation by computing the chart in this frame.

Formula $D_c = \frac{\text{mm.}}{1000} \times P^2$.

Rx	DISTANCE MOVED IN MM.	BECOMES	PRACTICAL Rx
Example: +12.00	13	1.87	1.87
A) +16.00	3	?	?
B) −14.00	4	?	?
C) +9.00 +1.00 × 90	5	?	?
D) −8.00 −2.00 × 180	6	?	?

Answer 1272. Continue . . .

Frame 1273. Plugging the solution into the formula:

O.D. $M_t = M_s \times M_p$

$$M_t = \frac{1}{1 - \frac{t \times D}{n}} \times \frac{1}{1 - D_v \times h}$$

$$M_t = \frac{1}{1 - \frac{(.0032 \times 8.25)}{1.523}} \times \frac{1}{1 - (2.5 \times .013)}$$

$$M_t = 1.0176 \times 1.0336$$

$$M_t = 1.0518$$

Magnification % = $(M_t - 1) \times (100)$
Magnification % = $(1.0518 - 1) \times 100$
Magnification % = 5.2%

Answer 859. **+3.75.**

Frame 860. The base curve formulas presented in this chapter are for glass lenses.

Because plastic is flatter than glass, base curves for plastic will have a number **(higher/lower)** than glass.

____

Answer 997. **None required.**

Frame 998.

VERTICAL DECENTRATION (+CYL)

	WHEN	DECENTRATION UP	DECENTRATION DOWN
B)	O.D. axis is between 90 and 180 O.S. axis is between 0 and 90	Induces △ Base In	Induces △ Base Out
	O.D. axis is between 0 and 90 O.S. axis is between 90 and 180	Induces △ Base Out	Induces △ Base In

Chart A is to be used for horizontal oblique axis decentration and Chart B is for vertical oblique axis decentration. The charts are for **(plus/minus)** cylinders only.

____

Answer 1135. See answers in next frame.

Frame 1136.

Rx	DISTANCE MOVED IN MM.	BECOMES	PRACTICAL Rx
A) +16.00	3	0.76	0.75
B) −14.00	4	0.78	0.75
C) +9.00 +1.00 × 90	5	0.40 × 90	0.50 × 90
		0.50 × 180	0.50 × 180
D) −8.00 −2.00 × 180	6	0.60 × 90	0.62 × 90
		0.38 × 180	0.37 × 180

Answer 1273. Continue . . .

Frame 1274.

O.S. $M_t = M_s \times M_p$

$$M_t = \frac{1}{1 - \dfrac{(t \times D)}{n}} \times \frac{1}{1 - D_v \times h}$$

$$M_t = \frac{1}{1 - \dfrac{(.0025 \times 6.50)}{1.523}} \times \frac{1}{1-(1.00 \times .013)}$$

$$M_t = 1.0108 \times 1.0132$$

$$M_t = 1.0241$$

$$\text{Magnification }\% = (M_t - 1) \times 100$$
$$= (1.0241 - 1) \times 100$$
$$= 2.4\%$$

If O.D. is 5.2% and O.S. is 2.4%, do you think the difference in magnification between the two eyes is **(2.8/7.4)**?

Answer 860. Lower.

Frame 861. Flatter base curves will have lower numbers. The base curve for a glass lens of −4.00 will be higher than a plastic lens of −4.00. A general rule of thumb is that plastic is approximately 1% flatter.

Base curves for plastic lenses are generally 1% **(steeper/flatter)** than glass lenses.

Answer 998. Plus.

Frame 999. The charts in Frames 997 and 998 can help the Optician predict and understand the Optical phenomena which occur as a Rx with oblique axis is decentered up or down, in or **(out/angled)**. The charts are prepared for plus cylinders only.

If minus cylinders are used, the Optician should logically **(invert/reverse)** all base directions.

Answer 1136. None required.

Frame 1137.

CHAPTER 17
LENS CLOCK

PLEASE CONTINUE TO THE TOP OF PAGE 212, **FRAME 1138**

Answer 1274. 2.8%.

Frame 1275. Now that you know that the magnification is manageable, that is, not beyond 5%, you can begin to balance the aniseikonia. Chapter 15 taught you the rules: Increase base curve and center thickness to increase magnification. Increase Vertex Distance in plus Rx's to increase magnification. You know you can compensate this Rx by increasing the magnification of the O.S. and decreasing the magnification of the O.D. Study the solution in this frame.

Rx	Base Curve	Thickness	Vertex
O.D. +2.50	+6.50	3.0 mm.	?
O.S. +1.00	+10.00	4.5 mm.	?

Answer 861. Flatter.

Frame 862. Opticians who indiscriminately demand specific base curves from the lab often wait for special or unusual bases to be ordered. The formula presented in this chapter is intended as a guideline only and not meant to be precise and fixed.

The formula presented by Vogel is designed as a **(hard and fast rule of optics/guideline).**

Answer 999. Out, reverse.

Frame 1000. Prismatic effects are induced as the eyes look through lenses at points other than the optical center.

The dispensing Optician can best perform the role of filling the prescription by fully understanding the consequences of **(decentration/concentration).**

Answer 1137. Go to Frame 1138.

Frame 1138. Opticians call the Lens Gauge by its optical nickname, The Lens Clock. The lens clock measures the radius of curvature of lenses. Study the illustration in this frame. The illustration shows the lens clock measuring the radius of curvature in diopters.

The clock is measuring the **(concave/convex)** surface of the lens and the dial is pointing to 6. Do you think this is **(plus/minus)** 6?

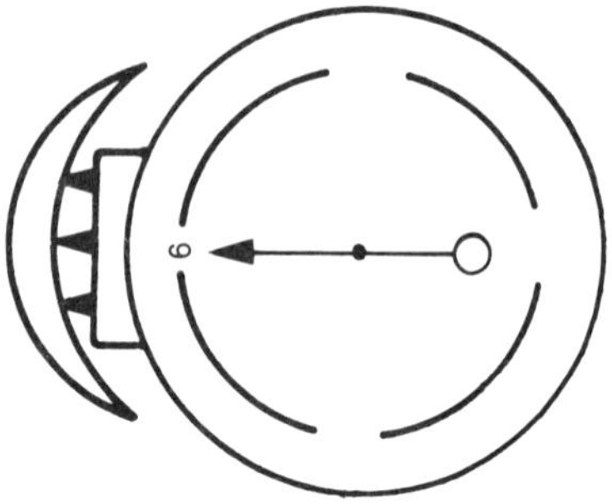

Answer 1275. Continue . . .

Frame 1276. Theoretically, you might wish to increase the vertex distance of the O.D. to increase magnification and at the same time, decrease the vertex distance of the O.S. However, this would be impractical since the frame would have to be distorted. The vertex distance, then, should be left alone at 13 mm.

If you re-calculate the new base curves and thickness, the resultant magnification difference will be seen to be reduced from 2.8% to less than 1%.

Comment: Management of aniseikonia drastically alters the magnification of lenses. Before undertaking the time-consuming mathematics, it is wise to estimate the chances for success.

Answer 862. Guideline.

Frame 863. The Optician thinks of base curves as a basis or beginning of lens design. Best base curve selection is predicated upon four dispensing rules: The difference in prescription power from the previous Rx and the new Rx, the present base curve, the difference between index of refraction of the material from the previous Rx to the present Rx, and the use of charts or formulae like Vogel's.

There are **(only/four)** major guidelines to correct base curve selection.

Answer 1000. Decentration. (Well, perhaps concentration, also!)

Frame 1001.

CHAPTER 13
MULTIFOCAL ANALYSIS

TURN TO THE BOTTOM OF PAGE 215, **FRAME 1002**

Answer 1138. Concave, minus.

Frame 1139. The lens clock can also be used to 'read' the prescription of single vision and some multifocal lenses. Study the example in this frame. The example shows a lens clock measuring the plus and minus side of the same lens.

The power of this lens is **(−1.00/+1.00)**.

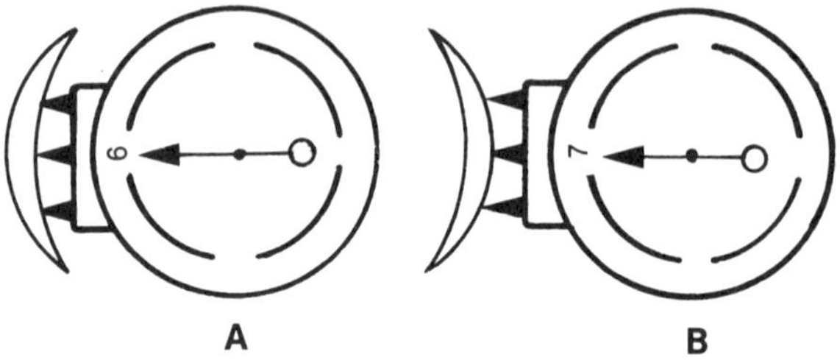

Answer 1276. Continue . . .

Frame 1277. Interaction with the doctor can prevent lots of hard work for little reward. In the case of cataracts and intraocular lenses, if the unoperated eye is to become aphakic soon, the doctor may wish you to hold off aniseikonic compensation.

Knowing that aniseikonic management produces unusual curves and thicknesses, if you find a patient wearing glasses like the ones illustrated in this frame, and the data shows:

Rx	Base Curve	Thickness
O.D. +5.00	+ 4.00	2.5
O.S. +1.50	+12.00	4.5

There is a possibility that these have **(been/not been)** compensated.

Answer 863. Four.

Frame 864. There are four major guidelines to best base curve selection. The correct choice of base curve is one which integrates the four guidelines, the doctor's preference, if stated, and above all, the patient.

The correct base curve depends upon **(many/one)** factor(s).

Answer 1001. None required.

Frame 1002. There are two major optical phenomena regarding multifocals. The first major phenomenon deals with the prismatic effect called, image displacement. Image displacement occurs as the eyes look through the lens vertically, from the distance lens down to the juncture of the bifocal segment.

Study the illustrations in this frame. The illustrations show the anatomy of a **(bifocal/trifocal)**.

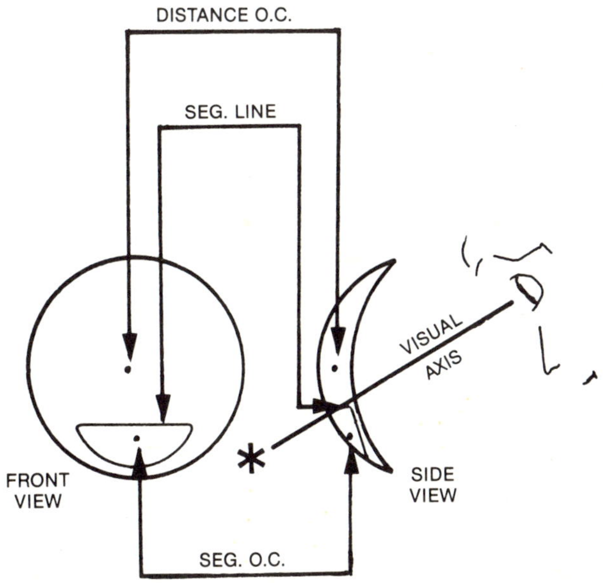

Answer 1139. +1.00 (−6.00) + (+7.00) = +1.00.

Frame 1140. The clock has two sets of scales: an outer scale for plus (black) and an inner scale for minus (red).* Study the illustration in this frame. The illustration shows a lens clock measuring **(+10.00/−14.00).**

*Although most lens clocks use red and black, some clocks use only black.

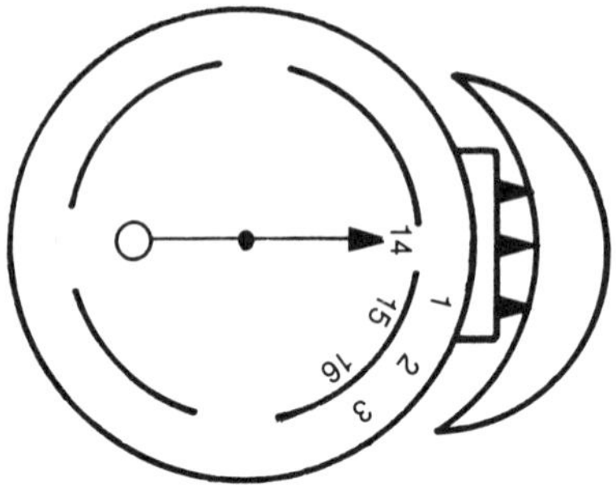

Answer 1277. Been.

Frame 1278. An unusual pair of glasses should cause the Optician to conclude they may have been changed **(purposely/carelessly)** and questions **(should/should not)** be asked.

Answer 864. Many.

Frame 865.

CHAPTER 7
THE OPTICAL CENTER

TURN TO THE TOP OF PAGE 218, **FRAME 866**

Answer 1002. Bifocal.

Frame 1003. As the line of sight crosses the juncture of the distance and the segment, a prismatic effect occurs. This image displacement causes the image to appear to "jump up" in front of the eye.

For this reason, Opticians call this image displacement **(jump/jump up)**.

Answer 1140. −14.00.

Frame 1141. When lenses are spherical, the algebraic sum of their convex and concave curves results in the lens power.

When lenses are compound, each meridian must be calculated **(together/separately)**.

Answer 1278. Purposely, should.

Frame 1279.

Title: **VERTEX VEXATIONS**

Situation: A good patient of yours tells you her mother is visiting from out of town and accidently stepped on her glasses. You are asked to duplicate them exactly. The data is as follows:

Data: Rx O.D. +13.50 +3.50 × 180
O. S. +14.75 +3.00 × 90
ADD +3.25
V.D. 8 mm.

Since this is a strong prescription, you ask the patient if she **(has/never had)** a copy of her Rx.

Answer 865. No answer required.

Frame 866. The optical center of a lens is defined as that point where light rays pass through undeviated. Study the example in this frame.

The illustration shows light rays passing through a lens.

The undeviated ray is **(A/B/C)**.

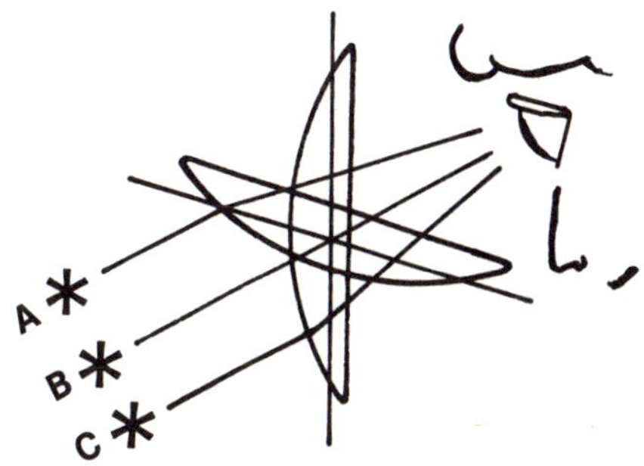

Answer 1003. Jump.

Frame 1004. Study the illustrations in this frame. The illustrations show two bifocal styles. The Rx for both lenses are:

O.D. PLANO
O. S. PLANO +2.00 ADD

As the eye travels through the distance portion, down to the segment juncture, the prismatic effect can be calculated as:

$$\Delta = \frac{d \times P}{10} = \frac{(4) \times (0.00)}{10} = \frac{0}{10} = 0.$$

Consequently, there **(is/is not)** a prismatic effect created by the distance portions.

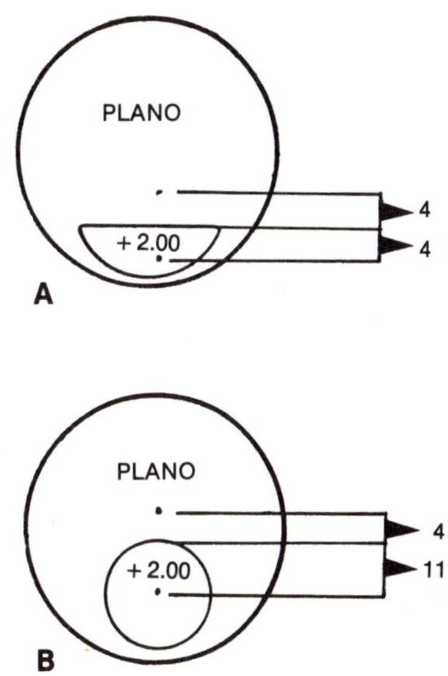

Answer 1141. Separately.

Frame 1142. Study the example in this frame. The front curve of this lens measured +8.50. The back curve measured −6.50 in the horizontal meridian and as shown in the vertical meridian. The optician can calculate the Rx by graphing meridians on an optical cross.

The Rx in minus cylinder is **(+2.00 −2.50 × 180/ +1.50 −3.00 × 180).**

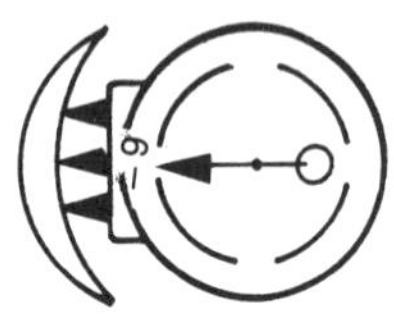

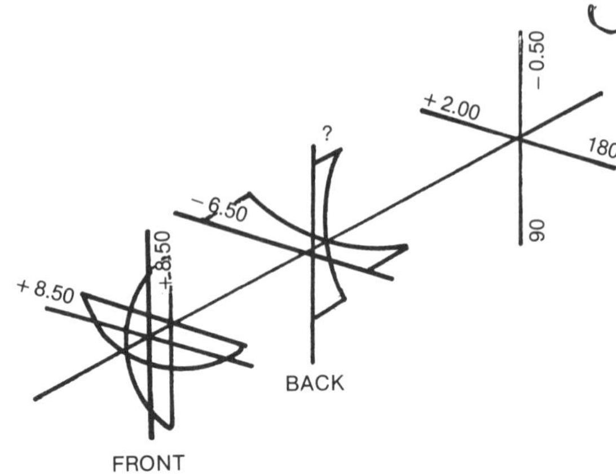

Answer 1279. Has.

Frame 1280. Fortunately, this wonderful woman was told by her Optician that carrying a copy of her Rx was a good idea and she produces it for you. The Rx reads:

O.D. +12.50 +3.00 × 180
O.S. +13.50 +2.50 × 90 V.D. = 14 mm.
ADD +3.25

You help her select an appropriate frame for aphakia which sits at 9 mm. vertex.

Question: 1. Were the old glasses compensated?
2. What is the correct power to now order?

Answer 866. B.

Frame 867. The undeviated ray in Frame 866 is ray B. A ray of light passing undeviated through a lens is said to pass through the optical center. It is the goal of the dispensing optician to position the lens in front of the eye so that the optical center is aligned with the visual line of sight.

Study the diagram in this frame.

Example **(A/B)** is correctly aligned.

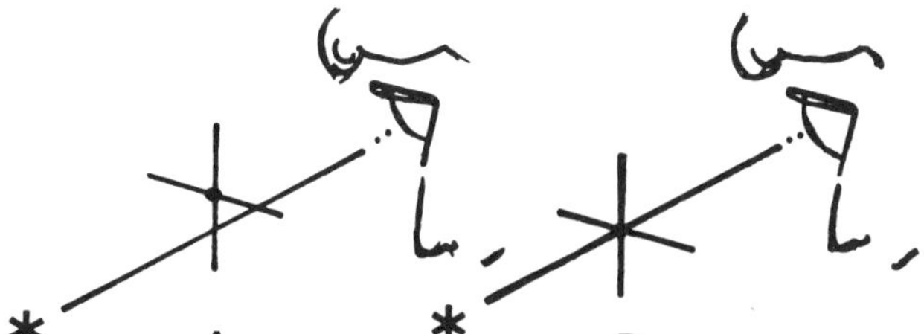

Answer 1004. Is not.

Frame 1005. Continue with the example in Frame 1004. As the eye encounters the segment juncture a prismatic effect occurs from the distance power **(+2.00/0.00)** and the seg power **(0.00/+2.00)**. For the flat top example, the distance between the seg center and the seg top is 4 mm. So, $\Delta = \frac{d \times P}{10} = \frac{(4) \times (+2.00)}{10} = 0.8\ \Delta$. For the Round Top Bifocal, the seg center is 11 mm. from the top, and the jump factor is $\frac{(11) \times (+2.00)}{10} = 2.2\ \Delta$.

From observation, then, you would think there is **(more/less)** 'jump' with the Round Top Bifocal than the Flat Top Bifocal.

Answer 1142. +2.00 −2.50 × 180.

Frame 1143. Reading prescriptions with a lens clock can be quite accurate (with the exception of the axis). Horizontal and vertical axis can be pretty well judged, however, oblique axis have to be guessed at.

Study the illustration in this frame.

The illustration shows a lens clock measuring the **(horizontal/vertical)** meridian in A and the **(horizontal/vertical)** meridian in B.

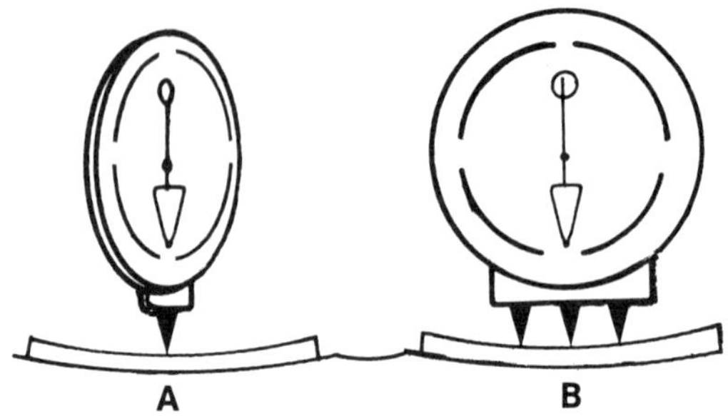

Answer 1280. None required.

Frame 1281.

Solution: 1. If the old glasses had not been compensated for, then the power would have been the same as the Rx copy. Therefore, the answer to question No. 1 is **(Yes/No)**.

2. The compensated power is found by calculating the focal length in each meridian, determining the new needed focal length and then converting back to realistic diopters for ordering.

First, work your own answers and then follow the steps in the next frame.

Answer 867. B.

Frame 868. B is correctly aligned. When light rays pass along the visual line of sight (the visual axis), directly through the optical center, the prescription is correctly aligned. Any mis-alignment of the optical center and/or the visual axis can cause unwanted optical effects.

Mis-alignment causes **(wanted/unwanted)** optical effects.

Answer 1005. 0.00, +2.00, more.

Frame 1006. The jump factor is greater for Plano distance with a +2.00 Addition for round top v.s. flat top bifocal.

Jump is determined by the power of the reading addition (seg), and the distance the top of the seg is from its optical center. Study the illustration in this frame.

Which lens has its O.C. closer to the seg line **(A/B)**?

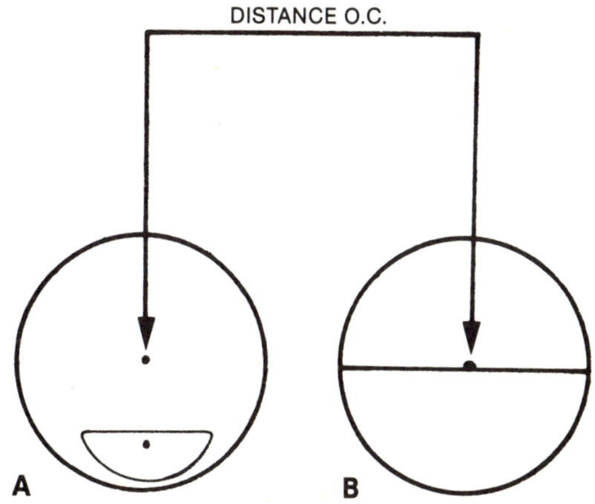

Answer 1143. Vertical, horizontal.

Frame 1144. The illustration in this frame shows the orientation of the principal axis. Illustration A is a view through the glasses as if you were wearing them and Illustration B is a view at someone who is wearing them.

Look at the examples once again. Two of the meridians are darker than the rest. If dark meridian #1 was −3.00 and dark meridian #2 was −4.75. This lens would have a **(cylinder/sphere)** power of **(−3.00/−1.75/−4.75).**

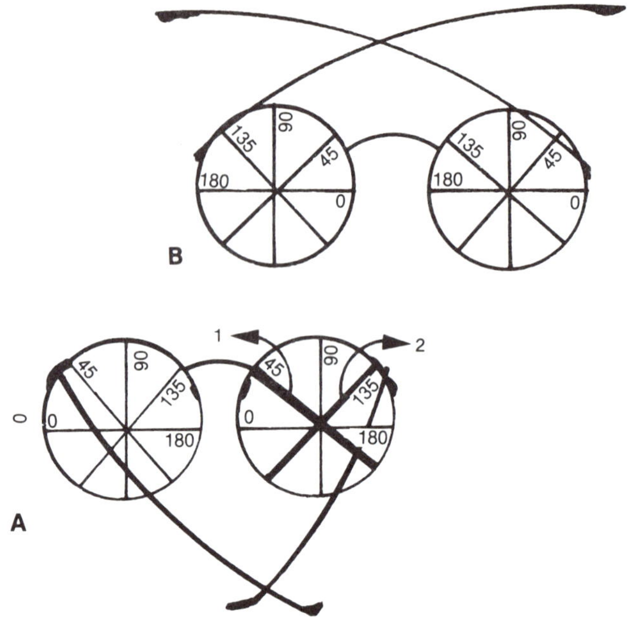

Answer 1281. Yes.

Frame 1282.

Horizontal:

Step 1. What is the focal length of +12.50?

$$f = \frac{1000}{D} = \frac{1000}{12.50} = 80.0 \text{ mm.}$$

Step 2. What lens is needed to focus 5 mm. less (14−9=5) than 80.0 mm.?
80.0 mm. −5.0 mm. = 75.0 mm.

Step 3. $D = \frac{1000}{f} = \frac{1000}{75.0} = 13.33 = 13.37$

Vertical:

Step 1. What is the focal length of +15.50?

$$f = \frac{1000}{D} = \frac{1000}{15.50} = 64.5 \text{ mm.}$$

Step 2. What is the needed focal length?
64.5 **(+/−)** 5?

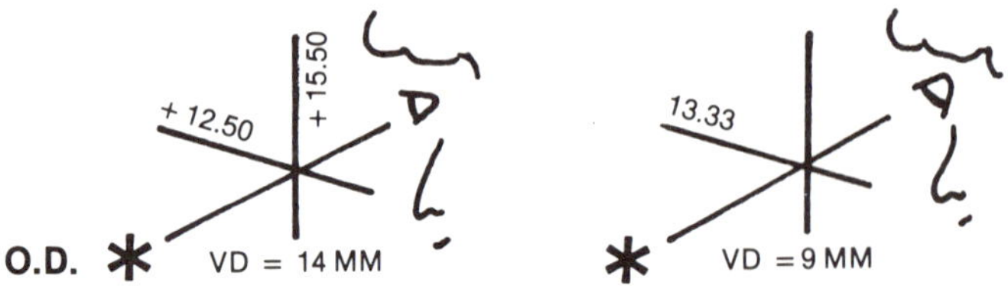

Answer 868. Unwanted.

Frame 869. One unwanted optical effect is called negative prism. Negative prism occurs as a result of the visual axis *not* coinciding with the optical center. Positive prism also exists. However, positive prism is prism created with a purpose. Positive prism will be discussed in another chapter.

There are **(one/two)** types of prism.

Answer 1006. B.

Frame 1007. A lens with its O.C. near or on the seg line will have less jump. As the visual line of sight crosses the seg line, the combined prismatic effect of 1) the distance power (P) times (×) the decentration (the amount of millimeters from the distance O.C. to the seg line) (d) *and* 2) the Add power (P) times the decentration (d) (the distance from the seg O.C. and the top of the seg), will equal the jump factor. Which equation do you think best illustrates jump? **(A/B)**

Distance and Add:

A) $J = \frac{(d \times P)}{(10)} + \frac{(d \times P)}{(10)}$

B) $J = \frac{(d \times P)}{(10)} \times \frac{(d \times P)}{(10)}$

Answer 1144. Cylinder, 1.75D. (Hold it! Before you look back, go on to the next frame below.)

Frame 1145. Now, think back to the last illustration without looking at it. If the base curve was +6.25 on the plus side and the lens clock showed −3.00 in dark meriian #1 and −4.75 in dark meridian #2, the Rx in minus cylinder form would be **(A/B)**?

A) +3.25 −1.75 × 45 B) +3.25 −1.75 × 135

Answer 1282. (−) Minus 5.

Frame 1283.

Step 3. 64.5 −5.0 = 59.5

$$D = \frac{1000}{f} = \frac{1000}{59.5} = 16.80$$

Step 4. Read the Rx in this frame:
+13.33 +3.47 × 180

Step 5. Round off for realistic ordering
+13.37 +3.50 × 180

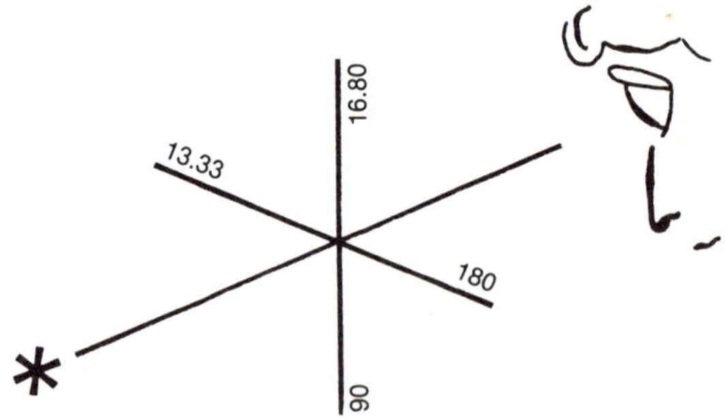

The Optician should order a practical O.D. +13.37 +3.50 × 180, Add **(+3.25/+2.25)**.

Answer 869. Two.

Frame 870. Negative prism occurs when the Optical Center is mis-aligned with the visual line of sight which passes directly through the pupil. The optical center is referred to by its optical nickname: The O.C.

By referring the O.C. to major reference points of the lenses, the Optician can direct the positioning of the **(O.C./oh see)**.

Answer 1007. A.

Frame 1008. The Jump Factor is of importance in the understanding of conventional multifocals.

Because the O.C. of the seg is further from seg top in round top or ultex than in flat top, the jump factor would be **(greater/lesser)**.

Answer 1145. +3.25 −1.75 × 45 (If you had difficulty with that, you need to review Chapter 2).

Frame 1146. Test your understanding of lens clock prescription reading by correctly completing the chart in this frame. Compare your answers with the correct ones in the answer section.

WHEN LENS CLOCK MEASURES	BASE CURVE ON PLUS SIDE	Rx =	IN MINUS CYLINDER FORM
Example: −2.00 × 90 −3.00 × 180	+8.50	=	−6.50 −1.00 × 90
A) −4.50 × 180 −2.00 × 90	+6.00	=	?
B) −7.00 × 45 −8.50 × 135	+4.50	=	?
C) −9.25 × 30 −6.25 × 120	+2.00	=	?
D) −10.00 × 90 −10.00 × 180	PLANO	=	?

Answer 1283. +3.25. The Add is included in the calculation.

Frame 1284. Now, let's do the O.S. +13.50 +2.50 × 90 ADD +3.25

Horizontal:

Step 1. What is the focal length of +16.00?

$$f = \frac{1000}{D} = \frac{1000}{16.00} = 62.5$$

Step 2. What is the needed focal length?
14 −9 = 5. 62.5 −5.0 = 57.5

Step 3. What is the power of 57.5 mm.?

$$D = \frac{1000}{f} = \frac{1000}{57.5} = 17.39D$$

Vertical:

Step 1. What is f? $f = \frac{1000}{f} = \frac{1000}{13.50} = 74.0$

Step 2. What is needed f? 74.0 −5.0 = 69.0

Step 3. What is D? $D = \frac{1000}{f} = \frac{1000}{69.0} = 14.49$

Step 4. Read the Rx in Illustration B.
+14.49 +2.90 × 90

The lab order should be +14.50 +3.00 × 90
Add +3.25

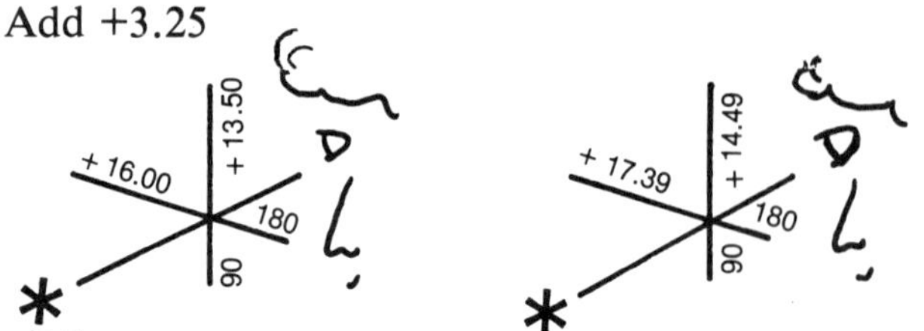

A O.S. + 13.50 + 2.50 × 90
+ 3.25 ADD
B

Answer 870. O.C..

Frame 871. Study the diagram in this frame. The diagram shows a boxed lens measurement of 52 × 42. The 'A' measurement is **(52/42)** and the 'B' measurement is **(42/52)**. The geometric center is $\frac{B}{2}$ or **(21/42)**.

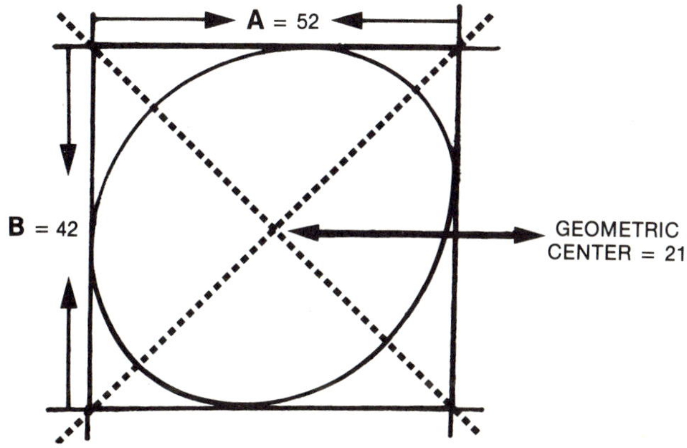

If the Optician wishes the optical center to sit 2 mm. higher than the geometric center of the lens, the lens is ordered as O.C. 2 above.

Answer 1008. Greater.

Frame 1009. Flat top bifocals provide less jump than round top lenses for minus prescriptions.

Which lens do you think provides less prismatic jump for plus lenses? **(Round top/Flat top)**

Answer 1146. **A) +4.00 −2.50 × 90 B) −2.50 −1.50 × 45 C) −4.25 −3.00 × 120 D) −10.00 sphere**

Frame 1147. Back in Frame 1139, Lens Clocks were said to be used to 'read' single vision and some multifocal lenses. Actually, lens clocks can only read solid bifocals rather than fused or bifocals inside the lens. Study the illustrations in this frame. The illustrations show bifocal A inside the lens, and bifocal B outside the lens.

Which lens looks like it is fused? **(A/B)**

Answer 1284. **None required.**

Frame 1285. *Comment:* When compensating for vertex distance, care must be taken to watch for changes in tilt, also.

For every 2° of pantoscopic tilt, the Optician should **(raise/lower)** the O.C. 1 mm.

Answer 871. **A = 52, B = 42, C = 21.**

Frame 872. By referring the O.C. to a major reference point, the Optician can direct the lab to correctly align the O.C. with the visual axis and thus prevent **(positive/negative)** prism.

Answer 1009. **Round top.**

Frame 1010. Plus lenses provide less jump in round top than in flat top. Consider the data below. A patient never wore glasses previously and the Optician wished to keep jump to a minimum. The Rx is

O.D. +1.00 Sphere
O.S. +1.25 Sphere
Add +1.50

The lens you would choose to minimize jump would be **(flat top/round top)**?

Answer 1147. B.

. . . .

Frame 1148. Solid bifocals are bifocals made of one piece. Study the illustrations in this frame. The illustration shows both a front and side view of the lens.

Which do you think is *not* a solid bifocal? **(A/B/C/D)**. You may choose two.

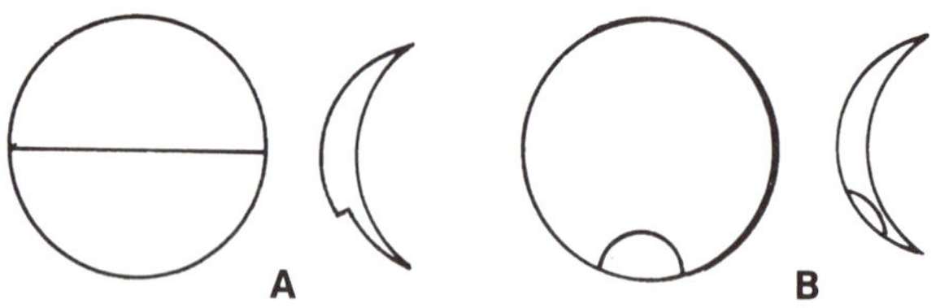

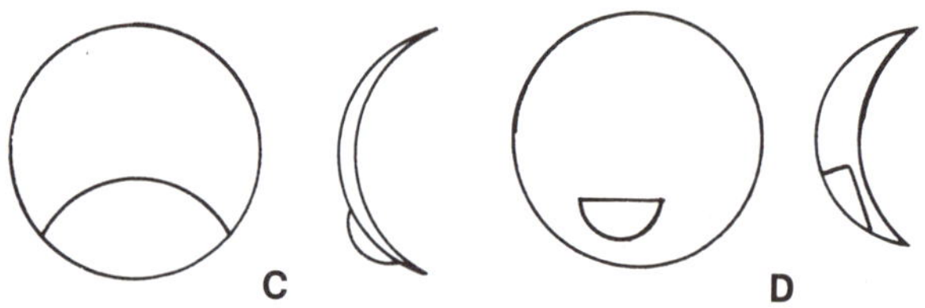

Answer 1285. Lower. See Chapter 16, Vertex Distance.

. . . .

Frame 1286. The Deadly Rx Chapter has shown that prime attention must be paid to the prescription to prevent it from "turning on you." This attention to prescription can be reduced to a routine which this author calls the Four A's of Dispensing.

The Four A's are:

ANALYZE
ASSESS
ASK
ADVISE

If you follow them, your chances for dispensing success will **(increase/decrease)**.

Answer 872. Negative.

Frame 873.

CHAPTER 8
DECENTRATION

TURN TO **FRAME 874**, AT THE TOP OF PAGE 235

Answer 1010. Round top.

Frame 1011. Some multifocals have little or no jump whatsoever, such as straight across (executive) and blended bifocals. Jump is of importance to the dispensing Optician in the understanding how lenses work.

Since most visual tasks involve the use of either the distance or the add, the juncture of the seg top and distance is of importance mostly for understanding the effect of round top or **(progressive/flat top)** multifocals.

Answer 1148. B and D.

Frame 1149. Only solid, one-piece bifocals can be read with a lens clock. The distance Rx is read like single vision lens, that is, the front curve (usually, the base curve), and the back curve values are added together.

The Add is determined as the difference between the distance and the seg readings. Study the diagram in this frame.

The diagram shows two lens clocks each with a different reading. The Add of this lens is **(+6.00/+8.00/+2.00)**.

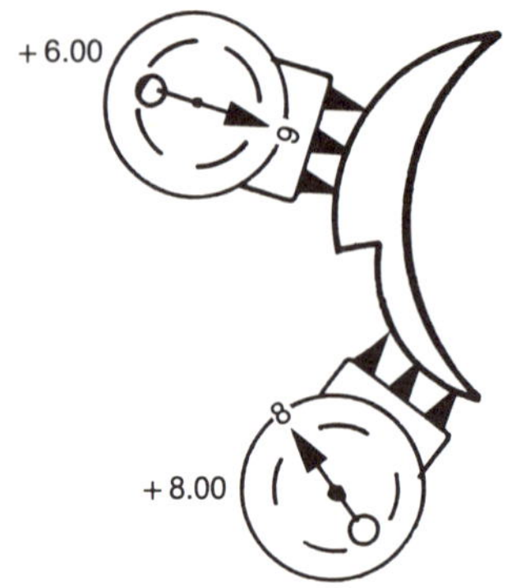

Answer 1286. Increase.

Frame 1287.

CHAPTER 24
OPTICAL FAIRY TALES
(And Other Fun Problems)

TURN TO THE BOTTOM OF PAGE 236, **FRAME 1288**

Answer 873. No answer needed.

Frame 874. The Optician decenters the lens to position the optical center directly in front of the pupil. This decentration may be placed (ground) in the lens by the laboratory optician, or it may be created by physically moving the lens center.

Study the illustration in this frame. The lens which has been moved off center (decentered) is **(A/B)**.

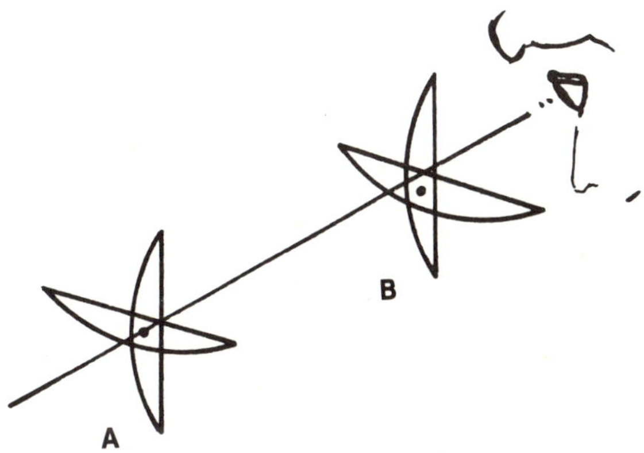

Answer 1011. Flat top.

Frame 1012. Back in Frame 1002, two major optical phenomena regarding multifocals was stated. One is image displacement or **(junk/jump)** and the other is object displacement. Object displacement is the prismatic effect which occurs as the combined optical effects of the distance Rx and the Add meet at some point for reading. Study the diagram in this frame.

The diagram shows the point of the visual axis as the patient is **(watching TV/reading)**.

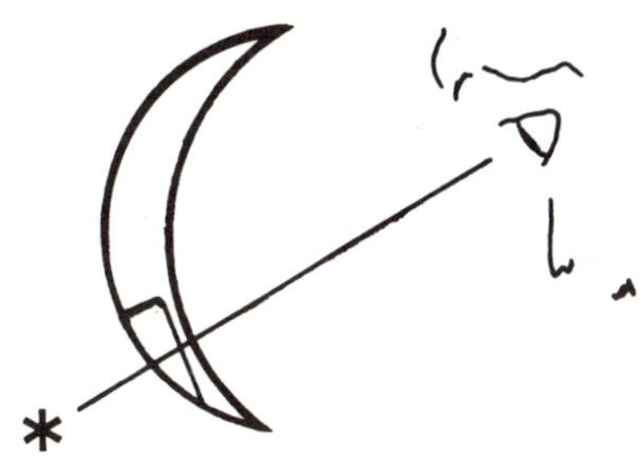

Answer 1149. +2.00.

Frame 1150. The difference between the reading of the segment and the distance equals the power of the Add. The distance reading, however, must be on the same side that the Add is on. Study the illustration in this frame. Which illustrations are correct? **(A/B/C/D)**

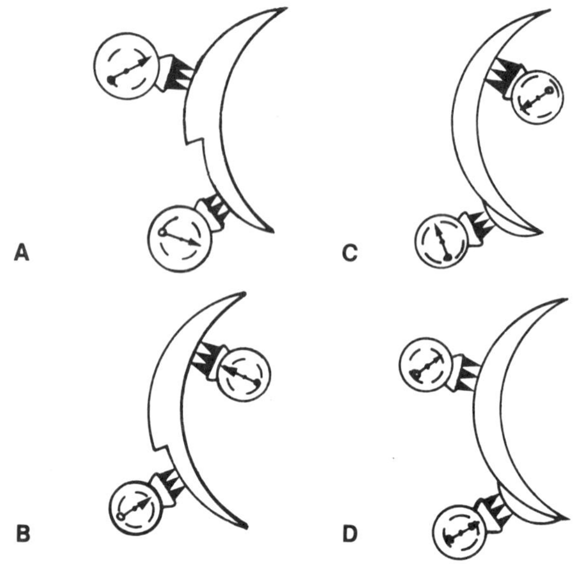

Answer 1288. None required.

Frame 1289.

THE RESOURCEFUL OPTICIAN

It is a cold, dark, rainy day and not one customer has walked through the door of Ophaxis Optical Company. The phone rings and Dr. Rhee Chek asks Ms. Dee Spencer if she could please check out a pair of glasses for him and give the patient a copy. Upon the patient's arrival, Dee turns on the lensometer only to find the bulb has blown and after a panic search, her worst fears are confirmed; no bulbs. Dee looks at the glasses. Photogray Executive Bifocals. She now knows that she **(can/cannot)** read the lens with a lens clock.

Answer 874. B.

. . . .

Frame 875. Decentration may be horizontal or it may be vertical. The Optician uses decentration in the placement of the optical center as a single point called the major reference point (M.R.P.).

Study the illustration in this frame. The M.R.P. must be located **(in/out)** and **(up/down)**.

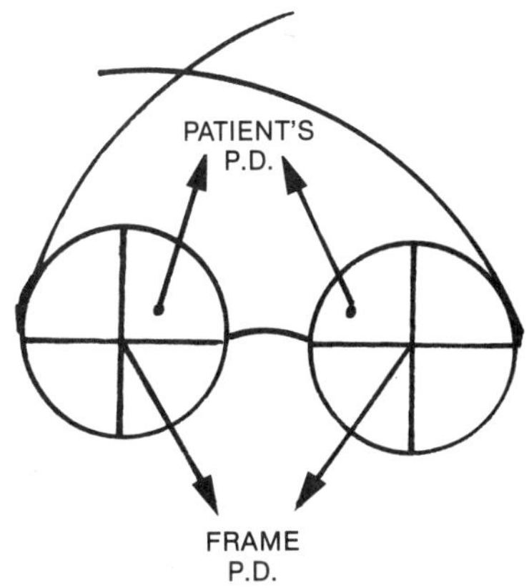

____

Answer 1012. Jump, reading.

. . . .

Frame 1013. A bifocal may be thought of as two separate lenses combined together. Study the example in this frame. The example illustrates two lenses with **(one/two)** optical centers.

The illustration shows the visual line of sight looking through the **(distance/add/both)** lenses simultaneously.

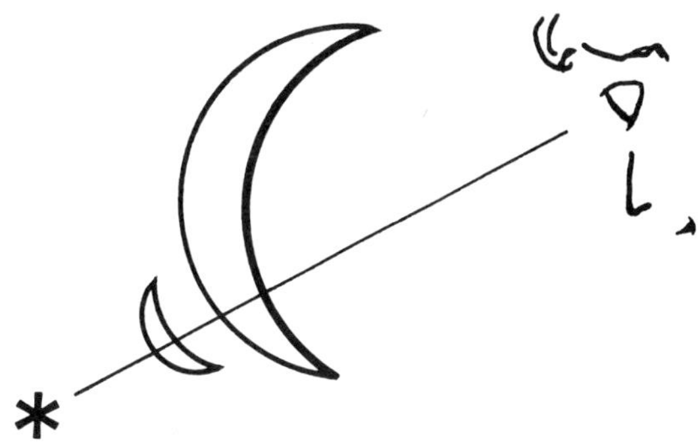

____

Answer 1150. A and D.

Frame 1151. Determine the prescription and Add from the illustrations in this frame.

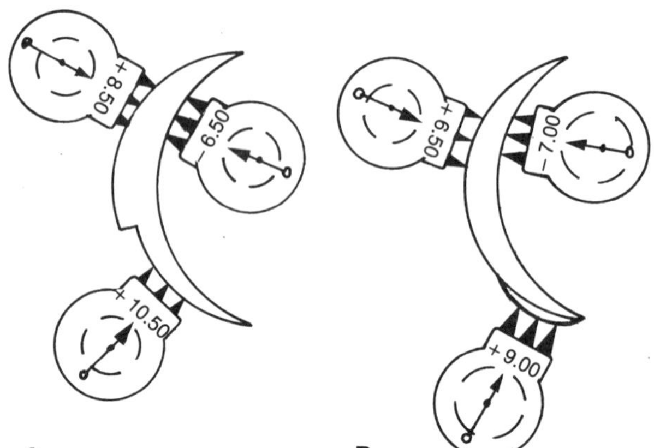

A B

Answer 1288. Can.

Frame 1289. Dee confidently measures the lens.

O.D. Front Curve +8.50
Back Curve −6.50 × 180 and −5.50 × 90

The segment measures +10.75.

Dee knows that the base curve is **(+2.25/+8.50)** and the Add is **(+10.75/+2.25)**. The Rx in the horizontal meridian is **(+2.00/−2.00)** and in the vertical meridian it is **(+3.00/−3.00)**. Because Dr. Rhee Chek writes his Rx's in minus cylinder form, the prescription Dee writes is **(+3.00 −1.00 × 180/ +3.00−1.00 × 090)**.

Answer 875. Up & in.

Frame 876. The amount of horizontal decentration is measured in millimeters and is calculated by subtracting the P.D. (pupillary distance) from the sum of dbl and boxed horizontal eye size. Horizontal decentration = (boxed horizontal eye size + distance between lenses [dbl]) − (PD).

Study the illustration in this frame. The boxed eye size is the **(A/B)** measurement.

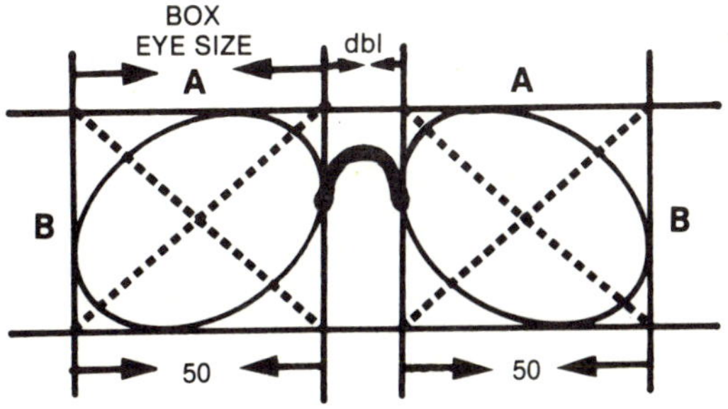

Answer 1013. Two, both.

Frame 1014. As the visual line of sight lowers itself through the distance portion of the lens and passes below the distance O.C., a prismatic effect is created as if the visual line of sight was looking through a prism whose base direction was either up or down. Study the diagram in this frame. The diagram illustrates two positions.

The position demonstrating the eye looking through a prism whose base direction is down is **(A/B)**.

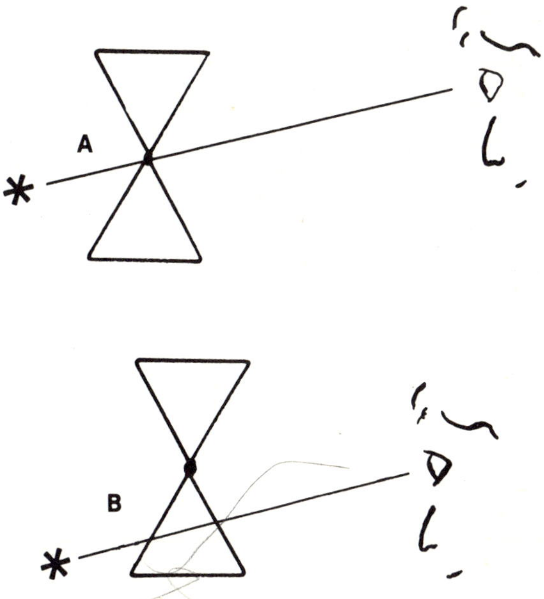

Answer 1151. **A) +2.00 Sph Add +2.00 B) −0.50 Sph Add +2.50.**

. . . .

Frame 1152. Naturally, the Optician doesn't need three lens clocks to read a prescription. The Optician should first determine the Add, then proceed to determine the distance. Which do you think would be the most efficient steps? **(A/B/C)**

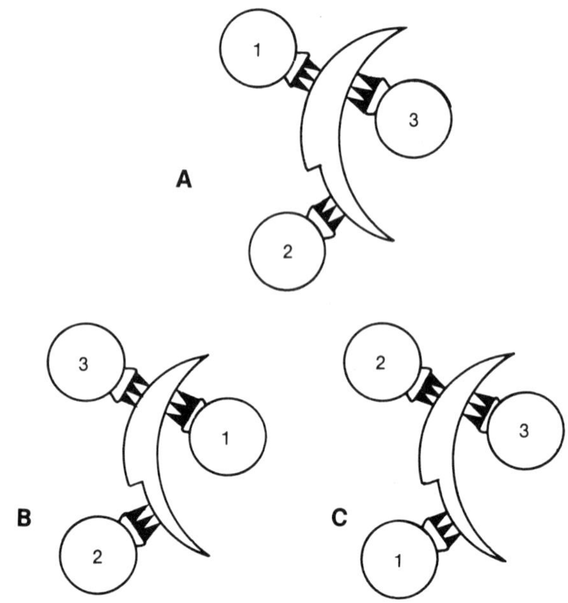

Answer 1289. **+8.50, +2.25, +2.00, +3.00, +3.00 −1.00 × 090.**

. . . .

Frame 1290. The O.S. lens clocks +8.50 on the front surface with +10.75 in the segment. The back curve in the horizontal meridian is −7.25 and in the vertical it is −4.50. The Rx is **(+4.00 −1.75 × 90/ +4.00 −2.75 × 90)** Add **(+2.25/+2.50).** Ms. Spencer writes out the Rx confidently. The patient leaves. Dee looks out and smiles as the sunshine breaks through.

Answer 876. A.

Frame 877. The boxed eye size is called the A measurement. The boxing measurement is found by drawing a box around the desired lens shape. Study the illustration in this frame.

The A measurement is the **(horizontal/vertical)** and the B measurement is the **(vertical/oblique)** box size.

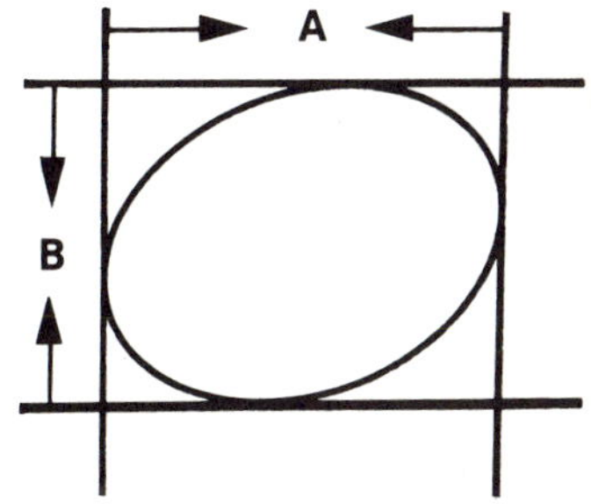

Answer 1014. B.

Frame 1015. Position B in Frame 1014 illustrates the lens visual line of sight looking **(above/below)** the distance O.C. Opticians reference the prismatic effect to the base of the prism.

Study the diagram in this frame. The diagram illustrates viewing through a prism whose base is **(up/down)**.

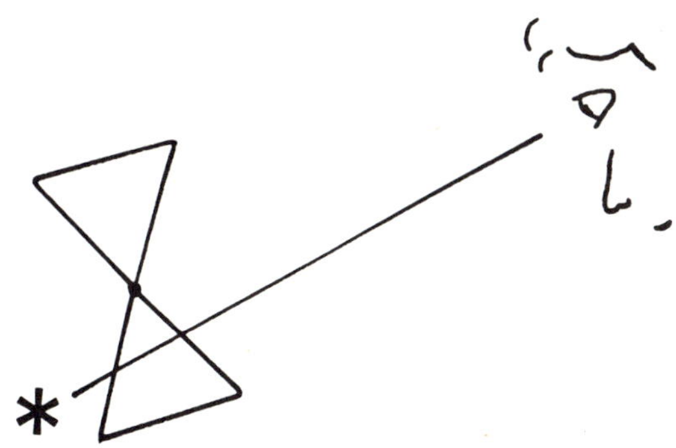

Answer 1152. C.

Frame 1153. Compound bifocal prescriptions follow the same rules of 'reading' as do single vision. Consider this problem. A lens clock reads an executive bifocal as +9.00 in the Add and +6.00 in the distance on the front surface. The back surface reads −8.00 at 180 and −6.00 at 90. What is the Rx in minus cylinder form.

The Optician **(can/cannot)** read this bifocal with a lens clock.

Answer 1290. +4.00 −2.75 × 90 Add +2.25.

Frame 1291.

THE FAMILY METROPIA

Miss Annie S. Metropia spoke little English. Both she and her Aunt had new Rx's. The ophthalmic dispenser looked dutifully at Annie's prescription:

O.D. −4.25 +2.50 × 45
O.S. −4.00 +3.00 × 180

Annie's job involved copying numbers from a screen, directly above her, on to narrow columns. Her eyes tracked vertically 10 mm. from the screen to the paper. This prescription **(has/does not have)** vertical imbalance for near and **(should/should not)** be compensatd for. The prismatic effect 10 below the O.D. has base **(down/up)** and the prismatic effect 10 below the O.S. has **(down/up)**. The amount of prism O.D. is **(______ diopters)** and O.S. is **(______ diopters)**. The correct method of compensating this Rx is to **(raise/lower)** the optic center in the **(O.D./O.S.)**.

Answer 877. Horizontal, vertical.

Frame 878. The A box measurement is horizontal and the B box measurement is vertical. The needed horizontal decentration equals the eyesize (A measurement) plus the dbl, minus the P.D. Study the illustration in this frame.

The dbl is represented by the letter **(X/A/B)**.

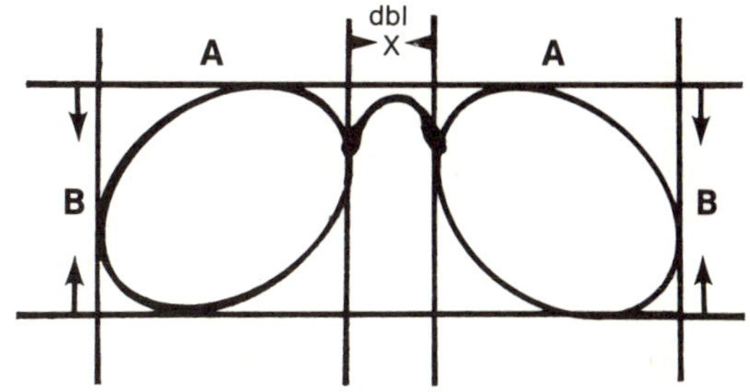

Answer 1015. Below, down.

Frame 1016. Because the prismatic effect is referred to the position of the prism base, the illustration of the prismatic effect in Frame 1015 is called base down. Study the example in this frame.

The example illustrates a visual line of sight viewing through a base **(up/down)** prism thus resulting in base **(up/down)** prismatic effect.

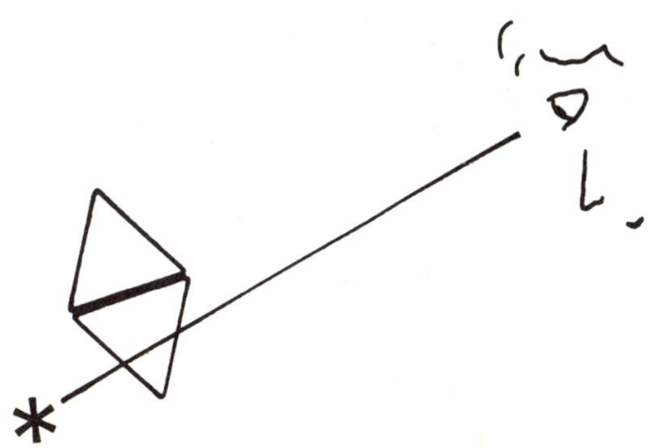

Answer 1153. Can.

Frame 1154. Here is the data once again. Solve the problem along with me.

	FRONT SURFACE	BACK SURFACE	READS
ADD	+9.00	−8.00 × 180	?
DISTANCE	+6.00	−6.00 × 90	?

Step 1. Add = (+9.00) − (+6.00) = +3.00

Step 2. Distance Base Curve = +6.00

Step 3. Plano −2.00 × 90 +3.00 ADD

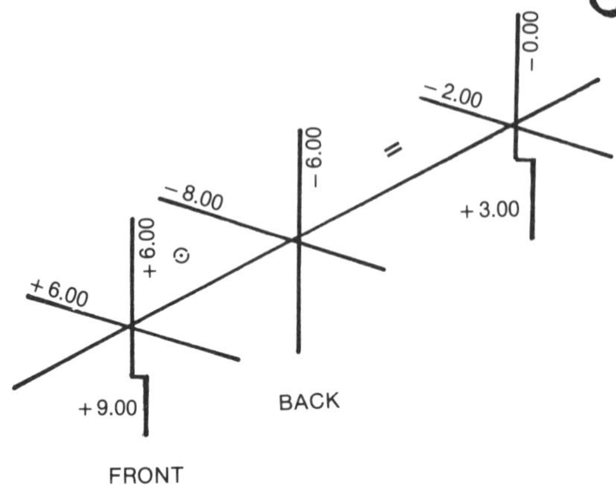

The cylinder on executive bifocals is ground in the **(front/back)** surface.

Answer 1291. Has, should, down, down, 3, 1, lower, O.D.

Frame 1292. Auntie Metropia had been wearing single vision lenses:

O.D. −1.00 −1.00 × 180 O.S. +3.00 −2.00 × 45

and now needed bifocals. Her new Rx increased only slightly for far:

O.D. −1.50 −1.50 × 180 O.S. +3.25 −2.50 × 45
ADD +2.00 Reading 8 below

Auntie Metropia **(will/will not)** have a problem for distance. She **(will/will not)** have a problem for near. The imbalance for near O.D. is (______ **D)** base **(up/down)** and O.S. (______ **D)** base **(up/down)**. The total imbalance is (______ **D)** base **(up/down) (O.D./O.S.)**.

Answer 878. X.

Frame 879. The dbl is the least distance between the lenses. Opticians refer to the dbl by its optical nickname: the bridge size.

The bridge size and dbl are the different names for the **(same/some)** thing.

Answer 1016. Up, up.

Frame 1017. In optics, plus lenses are considered to be two prisms whose "bases" touch and minus lenses are two prisms whose "apexes" touch. Study the illustration in this frame.

The minus lens is **(A/B)**?

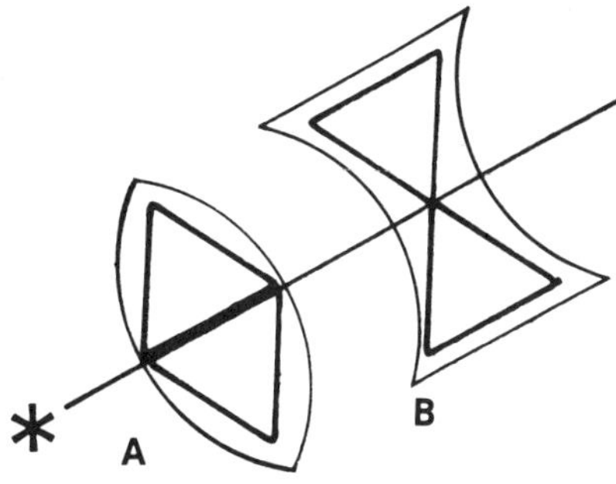

Answer 1154. Back.

Frame 1155. Test your ability to 'read' solid bifocals with a lens clock by solving the prescriptions in this frame. Give your answer in minus cylinder form.

		FRONT SURFACE	BACK SURFACE
A)	Add Reads	+8.50	−10.00 × 180
	Distance Reads	+6.25	−8.75 × 090
B)	Add Reads	+10.00	−10.00 × 180
	Distance Reads	+8.00	−4.00 × 090
C)	Add Reads	+2.25	−3.00 × 045
	Distance Reads	PLANO	−2.00 × 135
D)	Add Reads	+6.00	−4.50 × 120
	Distance Reads	+4.50	−4.50 × 030

Answer 1292. Will not, will, 2.4, B.D., 1.6 B.U., 4, B.D., O.D.

Frame 1293. Auntie Metropia's problem can be solved using **(three/five)** methods: ___________, ___________, ___________, ___________, ___________.

Which do you choose? ___________

Answer 879. Same.

Frame 880. The needed horizontal decentration is found by subtracting the P.D. from the sum of the A box measurement and the dbl. The sum of the eyesize and the bridge size (dbl) is equal to the frame P.D. Study the illustration in this frame.

The frame P.D. is **(70/50)**.

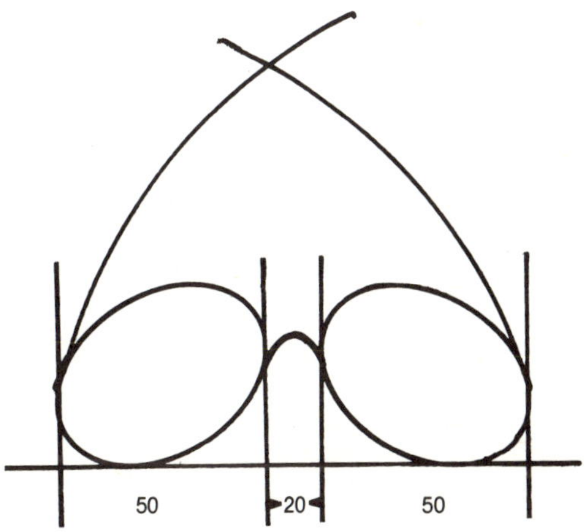

Answer 1017. B.

Frame 1018. The direction of the prismatic effect is determined by the direction of the prism base.

Match the illustrations on the right with the correct base directions on the left.

B.D.
B.U.
B.I.
B.O.

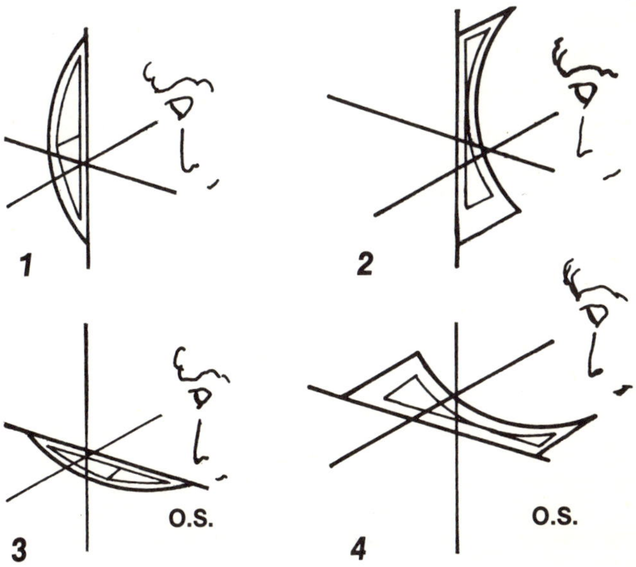

Answer 1155. **A) −2.50 −1.25 × 90 Add +2.25** **B) +4.00 −6.00 × 90 Add +2.00**
C) −2.00 −1.00 × 135 Add +2.25 **D) Plano Add +1.50**

Frame 1156. The lens clock provides the Optician with another tool for determining or verifying the prescription of a lens. Hand neutralization or Lensometry are other tools. For lenses with strong powers, special lens clocks exist.

Study the examples in this frame. The examples illustrate two lens clocks with **(similar/dissimilar)** 'feet.'

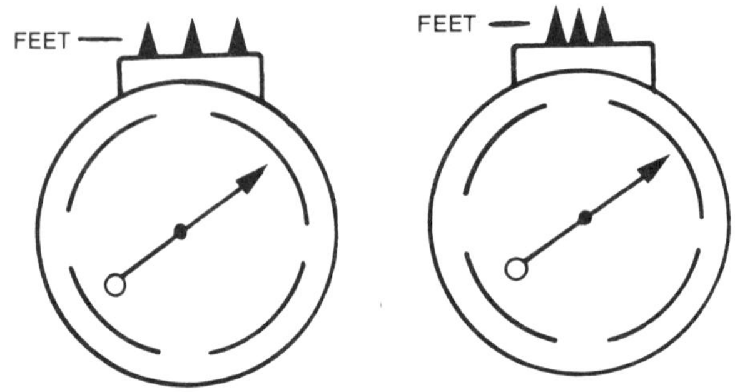

Answer 1293. **Slab Off, two pairs, prism segs, dissimilar segs, ribbon segs.**

Frame 1294.

THE THREE BALLS

Once upon a time, there were three Balls. Mama Ball (Mrs. I.), Papa Ball (Mr. I.), and Baby Ball (Odd). They all went to Dr. I.X. Ham for refractions.

Mr. I. Ball was a bilateral aphakic who needed little change in correction. His lenses were scratched, however, and Dr. Ham decided to give him a new Rx.

O.D. +12.50 −3.00 × 180
O.S. +14.00 −2.00 × 90 V.D. = 9 mm.
ADD +3.00

If the Vertex Distance is changed, then the effective power **(must/must not)** be altered.

Answer 880. **70.**

Frame 881. Horizontal decentration is found by subtracting the patient's P.D. from the frame P.D. If the patient's P.D. is 60 and the frame P.D. is 70, then the amount of needed decentration will be **(10/100)** millimeters.

Answer 1018. **1) B.U.** **2) B.D.** **3) B.O.** **4) B.I.**

Frame 1019. In multifocals, the combined lens effect of the distance Rx and the Add will equal the total prismatic effect. As long as the prescriptions in the vertical meridian remain somewhat similar, there is little binocular problem. When the eyes travel downwards through the lens to a reading position, the base down effect of minus and the base up effect of plus balance each other out. But, when the power is *not* similar, problems or discomfort can occur.

Dissimilar Rx's **(can/cannot)** cause problems of visual discomfort.

Answer 1156. Dissimilar.

Frame 1157. Special lens clocks for measuring strong powers have their 'feet' close together. Lens clocks which are used for plastic lenses also have special adaptation. Study the illustration in this frame.

From visual inspection alone, the lens clock that would cause the least damage to a plastic surface will have **(sharp/rounded)** feet.

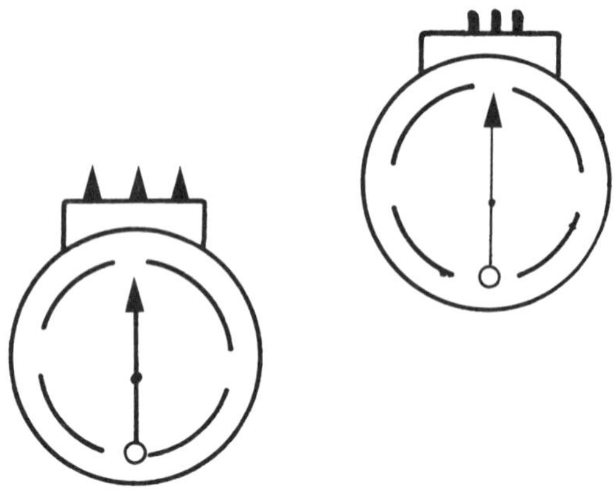

Answer 1294. Must.

Frame 1295. Mrs. I. Ball is myopic. Her new Rx is:

O.D. −3.00 −1.00 × 45 2 △ B.I.
O.S. −2.50 −1.50 × 135 1 △ B.D.

Odd Ball's Rx was:

O.D. +2.00 −4.00 × 180
O.S. +3.00 −2.75 × 90

The family takes their prescriptions to Ophaxis Optical Co. because their next door neighbor, Ann A. Apprentice works there. Ann first helps Mr. Ball as the others begin to try on frames. Mr. Ball decides on a nice combination frame which sits at a 12 mm. Vertex Distance, therefore, this Rx **(requires/does not require)** compensation.

Answer 881. **10 mm.**

Frame 882. The needed decentration in millimeters is ten. Since each lens must be decentered separately, the resultant decentration must be divided in half. Which do you suppose is the correct formula for decentration? **(A/B).**

A) $\frac{(\text{Eyesize}+\text{dbl}) - (\text{P.D.})}{2}$

B) $(\text{Eyesize}+\text{dbl}) - (\text{P.D.})$

Answer 1019. **Can.**

Frame 1020. A dissimilarity in the vertical meridian of multifocals can cause prismatic problems. When there is a significant difference in the vertical meridians of lenses, the object displacement at a given point for reading causes images to separate.

Significant differences in object displacement can cause **(separation/reparation)** of the image.

Answer 1157. Rounded.

Frame 1158. As valuable as lens clocks are to the Optician, they have one major drawback: Lens clocks are calibrated only for radius of curvature of crown glass lenses. Read the short Optical Fairy Tale in this frame:

"Once upon a time, there was only glass, whose index of refraction was 1.530. As the industry expanded and mass production began, the type of glass that was available in great quantity had an index of 1.523. So, the manufacturers of tools adapted or compensated for the difference.

Thus, today, the lens clock remains calibrated for **(1.523/1.530).**

Answer 1295. Requires.

Frame 1296. Ann looks carefully at Mr. Ball's Rx once again:

O.D. +12.50 −3.00 × 180
O.S. +14.00 −2.00 × 90 V.D. = 9 mm.
ADD +3.00

Ann knows that the vertex distance has **(increased/decreased)** with the new frame. This means the effective power has become **(stronger/weaker)** and compensating **(plus/minus)** has to be added. She remembers the short cut formula from W.A. Borover's book which calculates the effective power change as $D_c = \frac{\text{mmm.}}{1000} \times P^2$ where the change equals the distance (millimeters of movement) times the square of the power. Ann uses her calculator and first finds the horizontal axis. $D_c = \frac{\text{mmm.}}{1000} \times P^2 = (\frac{3}{1000}) \times (12.50^2) = 0.46$ or 050. This means that the horizontal meridian has to have 0.50 **(less/more)** power.

Answer 882. **A)** $\frac{\textbf{(Eyesize+dbl)} - \textbf{(P.D.)}}{2}$**, of course!**

Frame 883. The formula for horizontal decentration is (Eyesize+dbl) − (P.D.) divided by 2.

If the patient's P.D. is 72 and the frame P.D. is 70, then the needed decentration for each eye will be **(2/1).**

Answer 1020. **Separation.**

Frame 1021. The separation of images caused by a significant difference of power in the vertical meridians of multifocals when the eyes are in the reading position, is called 'anisometropia.' The word Aniso means "unequal" and metropia means "turning."

Therefore, anisometropia must mean an **(equal/unequal)** turning through lenses.

Answer 1158. 1.530.

Frame 1159. When materials other than 1.530 is to be 'read' using a lens clock, a conversion formula may be used to yield the true power. Because it is the true power for which the formula is used, the formula is called the **(flu power/true power)** formula. Study the illustration in this frame.

The illustration shows the anatomy of the true power formula.

$\frac{T}{D} = \frac{n - 1}{.530}$ where

T = True Power

D = Dioptric Power as measured by lens clock

n = index of refraction

Answer 1296. Increased, stronger, minus, less.

Frame 1297. Ann now continues with the O.D. and calculates the vertical meridian $D_c = \frac{mmm.}{1000} \times P^2 = \frac{3}{1000} \times (9.50^2) = 0.27$ or 0.25. Pleased with herself, Ann confidently does the O.S. Horizontal first:

$\frac{3}{1000} \times (+12.00^2) = 0.43$ or 0.50 and then Vertical $\frac{3}{1000} \times (+14.00^2) = 0.58$ or 0.62.

This Rx is represented in the illustration in this frame. Ann orders the correct compensated power from the lab as:

	Sphere	Cylinder	Axis
O.D.	?	?	180
O.S.	?	?	90
ADD +3.00			

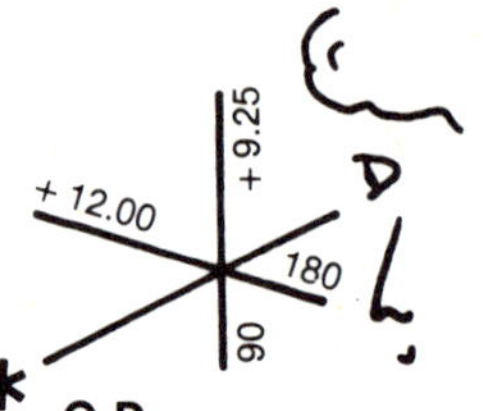

* O.D.

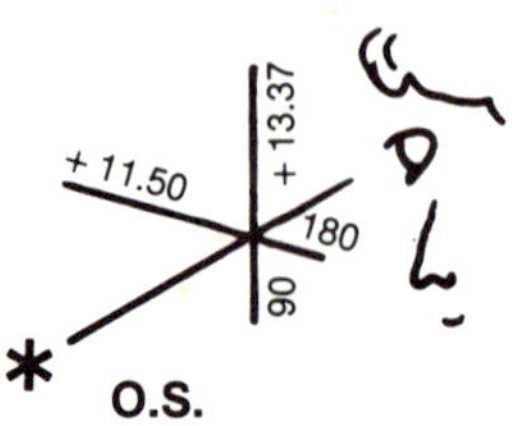

* O.S.

Answer 883. **1.**

Frame 884. Test your skill at determining the needed decentration for each eye from the information supplied.

Patient'sP.D.	Eyesize	dbl	Decentration
Ex: 64	52	18	3
A) 62	54	20	?
B) 70	50	16	?
C) 68	55	22	?

Answer 1021. **Unequal.**

Frame 1022. Opticians define anisometropia as an unequal difference between lens powers. As long as the visual line of sight passes through the distance optical centers, there is no prismatic effect. But, when the visual axis moves away from the distance optical center **(equal/unequal)** prismatic effects occur and can cause the patient visual discomfort.

Answer 1159. True power.

Frame 1160. The True Power Formula is a ratio proportion which is read "True Power is to Marked Power (lens clock), as the index of refraction of the material, minus one, is to .530."

OR $\frac{T}{D} = \frac{n - 1}{.530}$

If a lens clock 'reads' a plastic lens as +8.00, what is the True Power of the +8.00? n = 1.49

$$\frac{T}{D} = \frac{n - 1}{.530}$$

$$\frac{T}{8.00} = \frac{1.49 - 1}{.530}$$

$$\frac{T}{8.00} = \frac{.49}{.530}$$

$$T = 7.39 \text{ or } 7.40$$

Answer 1297. **O.D. +12.00 −2.75 × 180**
O.S. +13.37 −1.87 × 90 **ADD +3.00**

Frame 1298. Mrs. Ball's Rx once again is:

O.D. −3.00 −1.00 × 45 2 △ B.I.
O.S. −2.50 −1.50 × 135 1 △ B.D.

The frame she selected is a 52/18. The lens boxes 54 × 44 and her P.D. is 60. Ann knows that if she can use stock blanks (65 mm.) then she will save grinding prism charges. This Rx O.D. **(can/cannot)** be decentered enough to achieve 2 △ B.I. This Rx O.S. **(can/cannot) (either/also)**.

Answer 884. **A) 6,** **B) 2,** **C) 4.5.**

Frame 885. Opticians know that the human face is asymmetrical, or not perfectly formed. That is to say the P.D. must also be asymmetrical.

The distance between the center of the nose and the center of the pupil will **(always/seldom)** be the same.

Answer 1022. **Unequal.**

Frame 1023. When the visual line of sight passes through a point, below the optical center of the bifocal segment, the effect is as illustrated in this frame.

Do you think this is **(B.U./B.D.)**?

**HINT: Segs are Plus.

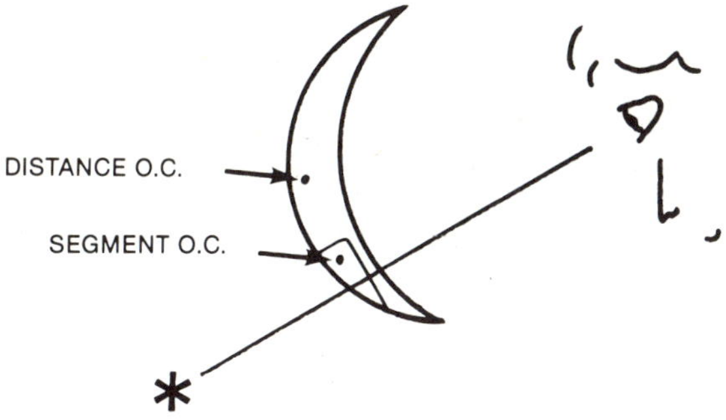

Answer 1160. None required.

Frame 1161. When compound lenses of material other than glass (1.523) are read with a lens clock, the Optician transposes each curve with the True Power formula and then proceeds with the true readings. Test your understanding of the True Power Formula by choosing the correct index of refraction for the formulas in this frame.

A) Glass $\frac{T}{D} = \frac{? - 1}{.530}$

B) Plastic $\frac{T}{D} = \frac{? - 1}{.530}$

C) Hilite $\frac{T}{D} = \frac{? - 1}{.530}$

$n = 1.49$
$n = 1.70$
$n = 1.53$
$n = 1.50$

Answer 1298. Can, can, also

Frame 1299. Mr. and Mrs. Ball's son, Odd, has been very patient. Actually, he was enjoying himself in the dispensary while Ann Apprentice was waiting on his folks. At last, it was his turn. Odd had already decided what he wanted: a big goggle shape like pilots wear. Ann looks at the Rx and data once again.

O.D. +2.00 −4.00 × 180
O.S. +3.00 −2.75 × 90
'A' Box = 56
'B' Box = 50
Dbl = 18
E.D. = 60
P.D. = 59

The frame sat very low on Odd's face, which meant he would be looking through a point 4 mm. above the distance O.C. Ann is certain that vertical imbalance **(will/will not)** exist.

Answer 885. Seldom.

Frame 886. In real life, the P.D.'s are seldom symmetrical.

Study the illustration in this frame. From visual inspection alone, the illustration shows **(symmetrical/asymmetrical)** P.D.'s.

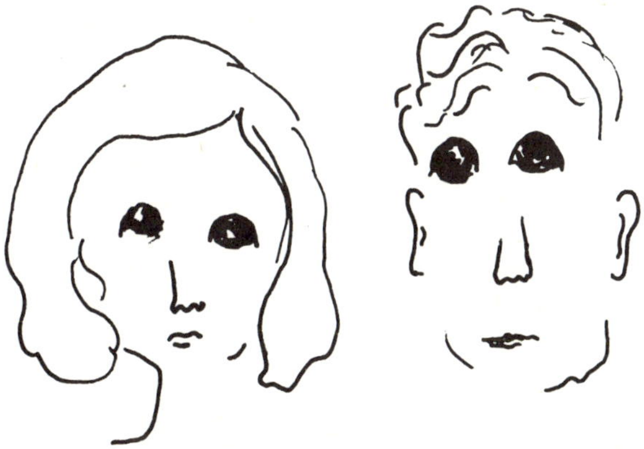

Answer 1023. B.U.

Frame 1024. When the visual line of sight passes through a point in the seg which is above the segment's O.C., then the effect is base **(down/up)**. When the visual line of sight passes directly through the optical center of the seg, there is **(some/zero)** prismatic effect. The Optician can determine the vertical prismatic effect of both the distance and the bifocal lens by calculating the total prismatic effect of the anisometropia. A simpler, usable method can also work.

There is another **(fusable/usable)** method.

Answer 1161. A) 1.53 B) 1.49 C) 1.70.

Frame 1162. The lens clock proves to be a valuable tool for determining or verifying lens powers. It is certainly easier to transport than a lensometer and in many cases, can be **(just/somewhat)** as accurate.

Answer 1299. Will.

Frame 1300. The prismatic vertical effect at 4 mm. above O.C. is **(0.2/2.0)** base **(up/down)** **(O.D./O.S.)** and if the visual line of sight remains at that point, Odd may feel the effects of the prism, so Ann decides to compensate. She notates on the order form to raise the distance O.C.'s 4 mm. Odd wanted his glasses as fast as possible, so Ann checked her stock. Yes, she had a pair of 70 mm. As the Ball family leaves, Ann decides to stay and cut and edge Odd's glasses so she could surprise him by getting them even sooner. Besides, the lab optician, Len Grinder, was on vacation.

Answer 886. Asymmetrical.

Frame 887. The P.D. for the right eye plus the P.D. for the left eye is called the binocular P.D. The P.D. for each eye separately is called the monocular P.D.

Study the illustration in this frame. Lines **(C–D/A–B)** represent monocular P.D.'s.

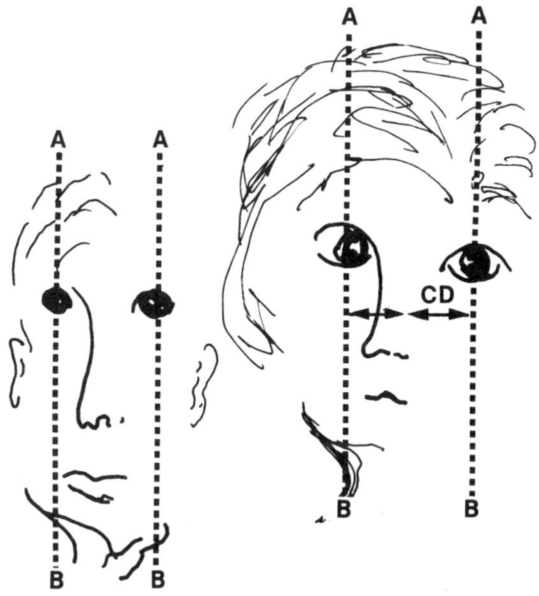

Answer 1024. Base down, zero, usable.

Frame 1025. The vertical prismatic effect (anisometropia) can be identified by multiplying the difference (in the vertical meridians) between the O.D. and O.S. times (×) the distance the eyes travel downward to read. Study the Rx and data in this frame.

O.D. −4.00 Sph
O.S. −1.00 Sph Add +2.00
Reading Level 8 mm. below the distance O.C.

The difference between the O.D. and O.S. is **(−3.00/−5.00).**

Answer 1162. Just.

Frame 1163.

CHAPTER 18
CUTTING AND EDGING

TURN TO THE TOP OF PAGE 264, **FRAME 1164**

Answer 1300. 2.0, B.D., O.S.

Frame 1301. Ann takes the O.D. first. She sets the axis wheel on the lensometer at **(90/180)** and the power wheel at **(+2.00/−2.00)**. Setting the lens in place, Ann slowly rotates the lens until the **(sphere/cylinder)** lines are sharp and clear and the lens is centered against the target. She then finds the cylinder. Inking the lenses, Ann marks the letter R with a grease pencil and carefully places it**(concave/convex)** side down in the shop tray. She then sets the axis wheel for the O.S. at **(90/180)** and the power wheel at **(+3.00/−2.75)**.

Answer 887. **C − D.**

Frame 888. Because of facial asymmetry, Opticians find that monocular P.D.'s are more accurate than binocular P.D.'s. When decentration is to be calculated, it is more accurate to use **(binocular/ monocular)** P.D.'s.

Answer 1025. **−3.00.**

Frame 1026. Follow the calculation further.

$$\triangle = \frac{d \times P}{10} = \frac{(8) \times (-3.00)}{10} = 2.4$$

Since the visual line of sight is looking below the O.C. of a minus lens the effect is as if looking through a base **(up/down)** prism and is called base **(up/down)**. *See illustration.*

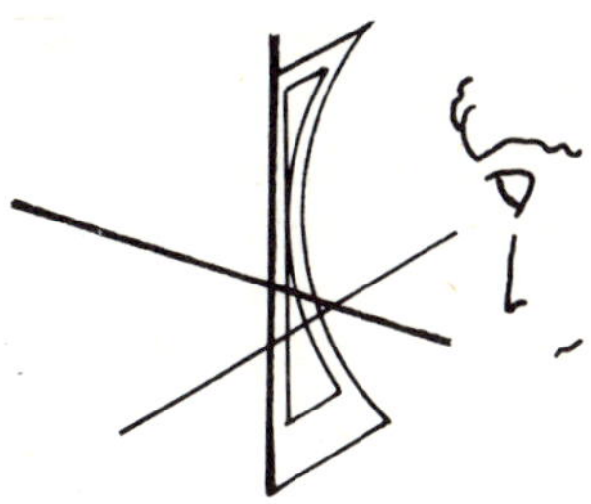

Answer 1163. None required.

Frame 1164. Opticians use the term 'cutting and edging' to refer to the process of positioning a finished lens blank and shaping it to fit a given frame. The term 'cutting' came from the days of Opticianry when a lens blank was scored (cut) with a glasscutter, then broken off (crimped), and left with a jagged edge. The term 'edging' came from the process of smoothing the edge against a stone. With the advent of modern edgers, the entire blank is 'edged' and shaped in one step.

So, cutting and edging, in the true sense, are really **(present/past)** processes.

Answer 1301. 180, +2.00, sphere, concave, 90, +3.00.

Frame 1302. After both lenses are spotted (inked), Ann places the right lens on a grid for the layout process. She centers the lens concave side toward her (up) and decenters the O.D. _______ mm. to the **(left/right)**, thus decentering **(in/out)**. As she looks at the order form, she recalls wanting to raise the O.C. 4 mm. so she also moves the center **(up/down)**.

Answer 888. Monocular.

Frame 889. As mentioned in Chapter 7, the decentration of the O.C. may be decentered, horizontal *or* vertical. If horizontal decentration is based upon the "A" box measurement, then vertical decentration must be based upon the **(B/C)** Box measurement.

Answer 1026. Down, down.

Frame 1027. When the Rx is compound, the vertical meridian must be used. Calculate the vertical prismatic effect of the following Rx.

O.D. +2.00 +1.00 × 180
O.S. +1.00 +2.00 × 90   ADD +3.25

Reading level 10 mm. below distance optical center.

Power in the vertical meridian
O.D. = **(+2.00/+3.00).**

Power in the vertical meridian
O.S. = **(+2.00/+1.00).**

Answer 1164. Past.

Frame 1165. Because the modern edger is equipped to bevel and shape the finished lens blank in one step, the process should really be called Shaping and Edging, but Opticians continue to use the 'nickname' Cuttin' and Edgin'.

The beginning of the shaping and edging process is the positioning of the Major Reference Points of the lens. Opticians call this positioning of the MRP "Layout." 'Layout' begins at the lensometer with the location of the Optical Center.

MRP's, OC's and Lensometry **(play/do not play)** a role in Layout.

Answer 1302. 7.5 mm., left, in, up.

Frame 1303. Ann now moves the O.S. **(7/7.5)** mm. to the **(left/right)** and **(raises/lowers)** the center **(4/0)** mm.

The pattern measures 41.5 mm. Ann computes the edger setting at **(51/31)**. The lenses were then edged and mounted. Ann performed verification by checking out the **(stronger/weaker)** lens first and thus selects the **(O.D./O.S.)**.

Answer 889. B.

Frame 890. "A" box measurement is used for horizontal decentration and "B" box measurement is used for vertical decentration. Study the illustration in this frame.

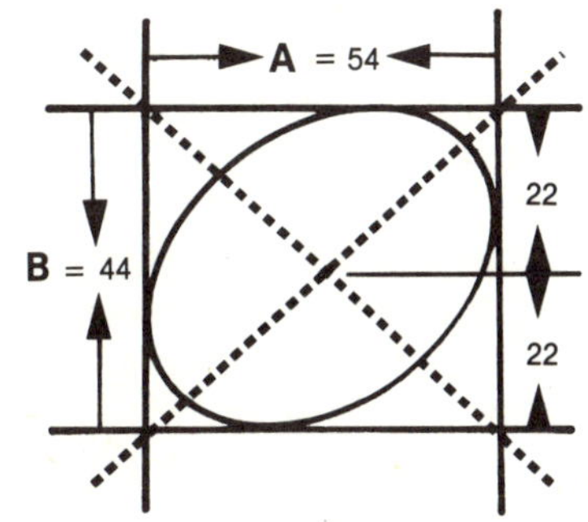

If the Optician requires the O.C. 25 mm. above the bottom of the lens, then the lens would require decentration in the **(upward/downward)** direction.

Answer 1027. +3.00, +1.00.

Frame 1028. The difference between the two lenses, then, is (+3.00) − (+1.00) = +2.00. Since the reading level is 10 mm., the equation becomes:

$$\Delta = \frac{d \times P}{10} = \frac{(10) \times (+2.00)}{10} = 2\,\Delta.$$

To determine the direction of the prism base, the Optician mentally visualizes the situation. Which do you think best illustrates this? **(A/B)**

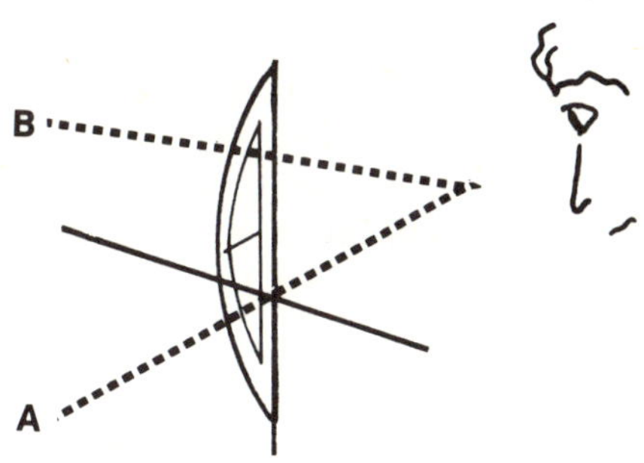

Answer 1165. Play.

Frame 1166. The Optician begins the Layout process by locating and marking the optical center (OC) of the lens.

Study the example in this frame. Illustration **(A/B)** shows a located and marked O.C.

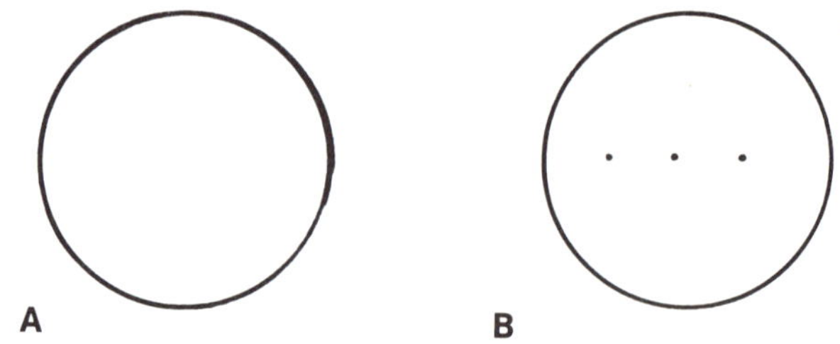

Answer 1303. 7.5, right, raises, 4, 51, stronger, O.S.

Frame 1304. Ann completed her verification. She was tired, but very proud of herself and anxiously waited Len's return so she could show her good work.

She closed the store that night with good feelings about Opticianry and wondered what the reaction would be when she called **(Odd/Even)** in the morning.

Answer 890. Upward.

Frame 891. If the "B" box measurement was 44 and the needed O.C. height was 25 mm., then the formula for needed vertical decentration would be "B" box measurement divided by two $\frac{B}{2}$ minus the needed height which is 25 mm. The formula is broken into two steps.

1) $\frac{B}{2}$ = vertical geometric center
2) Vertical Geometric Center − needed o.c. height = needed vertical decentration.

For the problem in this frame, then, the wanted O.C. height is **(25/52)**, the vertical geometric center is **(22/44)** and the "B" box is **(54/44)**.

Answer 1028. A.

Frame 1029. The prismatic effect of a visual line of sight viewing through a base up prism is base up, therefore, for the Rx in Frame 1028, the answer is 2 △ B.U. The greater power is in front of the **(O.D./O.S.)**, therefore, the prismatic effect is said to be 2 △ B.U. **(O.D./O.S.)**.

Answer 1166. B.

Frame 1167. Three dots (one on each side of the O.C. dot) placed by the lensometer spotting device produce a horizontal working axis line. For compound lenses, the Optician first sets the axis wheel of the lensometer, then places the lens in the holder of the lensometer. Study the Rx in this frame.

−3.00 +2.50 × 180

The Optician should first set the **(power/axis)** wheel at **(−3.00/180)**.

Answer 1304. Odd.

Frame 1305. You have now finished *Opticianry: The Practice and The Art — Volume II: The Science of Opticianry*. You have been through many concepts and exercises programmed to provide you a working knowledge of the prescription and its relationship to the patient. The next book in this series: *Volume III: The Dynamics of Dispensing*, will address the dispensing procedure itself.

Do you think *Volume III* will also be programmed? **(Yes/No)**

Answer 891. 25, 22, 44. If you missed any of these, review Chapter 6 & 7.

Frame 892. For a wanted O.C. height of 25 mm. when the "B" box is 44, the Optician uses the formula $\frac{\text{"B"}}{2} - 25$. One-half B box (44 ÷ 2) = 22, and 22 from 25 = 3. The needed decentration, therefore, is 3 millimeters and the direction is **(downward/upward).**

Answer 1029. O.D., O.D.

Frame 1030.

The Rx O.D. +2.00 +1.00 × 180
O.S. +1.00 +2.00 × 90 +3.25 Add

has a 2.4 Δ B.U. in front of O.D. as the visual line of sight passes through a point 8 mm. below the distance O.C.

In order to balance this anisometropia (vertical imbalance), the O.S. should also have **(2.4/4.2)** Δ B.U.

Answer 1167. Axis, 180.

Frame 1168. Once the lens is marked, the Optician decenters the horizontal and/or vertical positions as specified on the dispensing order form. Study the example and layout steps in this frame.

Rx O.D. = +3.00 −1.75 × 90
P.D. = 64
'A' Box = 52
Dbl = 18

Step 1. Set axis wheel at 90
Step 2. Insert lens.
Step 3. Rotate lens until Rx is centered and on axis. (Do not touch axis wheel.)
Step 4. Dot Lens.
Step 5. Decenter **(3/6)** mm. in.

Should you move center **(toward/away)** from nose of the O.D.?

Answer 1305. No. (Gotcha!)

Frame 1306. *Volume III: The Dynamics of Dispensing* will not be programmed. *The Dynamics of Dispensing* looks at the Psychology of the dispensing procedure, the words to say to prevent miscommunication. But beyond that, *Volume III* discusses the Optical Triangle.

Volume III discusses the dispensing procedure, as well as the Optical **(Rectangle/Triangle)**.

Answer 892. Upward.

Frame 893. Study the illustration in this frame, and compute the needed vertical decentration. The illustration shows a frame which sits high on the face. In order to avoid negative prism, the O.C. needs to be decentered **(downward/upward).**

The needed decentration then is: $(\frac{50}{2}) - 20 = 25.$

$25 - 20 = 5.$

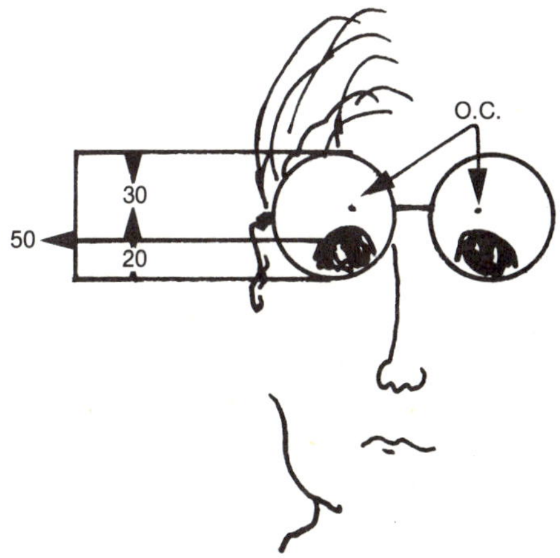

Answer 1030. 2.4 B.U.

Frame 1031. Multifocals, unlike single vision lenses, cannot have their optical centers manipulated in order to compensate for imbalances. The reason, of course, is that the seg would also be raised or lowered and become both cosmetically and optically unacceptable. Study the illustration in this frame.

Would you dispense a pair of glasses like those illustrated? **(Probably not/Yes/No)**

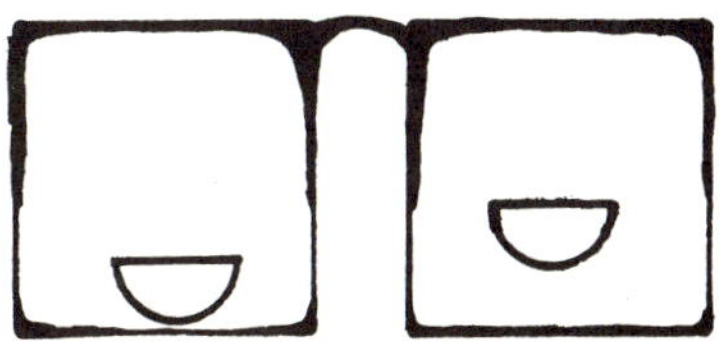

Answer 1168. 3, toward. (If you had any trouble with that, re-read the Chapter on Decentration.)

Frame 1169. A variety of marking devices exist, each with their own merits. Since the presentation of *all* of these devices are beyond the scope of this book, this author asks you to mentally picture a grid. The grid has increments of 1 mm. apart. Placing a spotted lens (no joke intended) on the grid will allow for correct decentration orientation.

Study the grid in this frame. The Grid shows a lens **(on/off)** center.

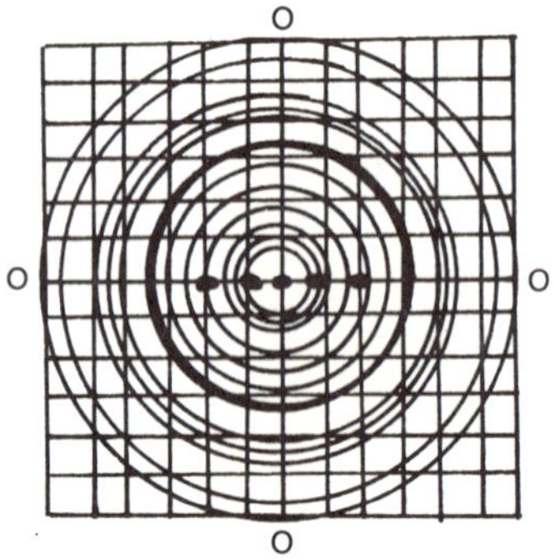

Answer 1306. Triangle.

Frame 1307. The Optical Triangle is the relationship between the Doctor, the Patient, and the Optician. When the relationship is good, all is well, when the relationship is poor, the Optician may find not only an unhappy Doctor, but an irate Patient, as well. *Volume III: The Dynamics of Dispensing* is also written to help develop a better you! I look forward to meeting you there.

Answer 893. Downward.

Frame 894. Test your knowledge of calculating the amount and the direction of the needed vertical decentration by correctly completing the chart in this frame.

	"B" box	Wanted O.C. Height	Decentration	Direction
Ex:	42	20	1 mm.	down
A)	46	25	?	?
B)	52	23	?	?
C)	57	26	?	?
D)	62	31	?	?

PLEASE TURN TO THE BOTTOM OF PAGE 1, **FRAME 895**

Answer 1031. Probably not.

Frame 1032. The methods of dealing with object displacement created by anisometropia continues in Chapter 14, but you have been working hard and deserve a treat. Turn to Frame 1033.

PLEASE TURN TO THE TOP OF PAGE 2, **FRAME 1033**

Answer 1169. On.

Frame 1170. Follow the layout steps for the following single vision lens.

O.S. Rx = +3.50 −1.50 × 150
P.D. = 62
'A' Box = 51
'B' Box = 40
Dbl = 19
O.C. = 22

Step 1. Set axis wheel at 150.
Step 2. Dot lens in lensometer. (See steps 1, 2, 3 in Frame 1168.)
Step 3. Decenter horizontal (51+19) − (62) = 8. 8 ÷ 2 = 4 in each eye.
Step 4. Decenter vertical $\frac{40}{2}$ = 20. 20 − 22 = 2.

Would you decenter the 2 mm. in Step 4 **(up/down)**?

PLEASE TURN TO THE BOTTOM OF PAGE 2, **FRAME 1171**

Answer 1307. See below.

Frame 1308. Place your order for *OPTICIANRY — The Practice and the Art: Vol. III, The Dynamics of Dispensing*, so that you can begin reading Chapter 1.

Gracie Enterprises, Inc.
P.O. Box 506
Chula Vista, California
92012-0506

APPENDIX

OBLIQUE AXIS CHART

AT DEGREES AWAY FROM AXIS			PERCENT OF POWER
0	OR	180	0
5		175	1
10		170	3
15		165	7
20		160	12
25		155	18
30		150	25
35		145	33
40		140	41
45		135	50
50		130	59
55		125	67
60		120	75
65		115	82
70		110	88
75		105	93
80		100	97
85		95	99
90		90	100

THIS CHART HELPS IN LOCATING ONE SPECIFIC FRAME

To find the frame number for a specific subject, see INDEX.

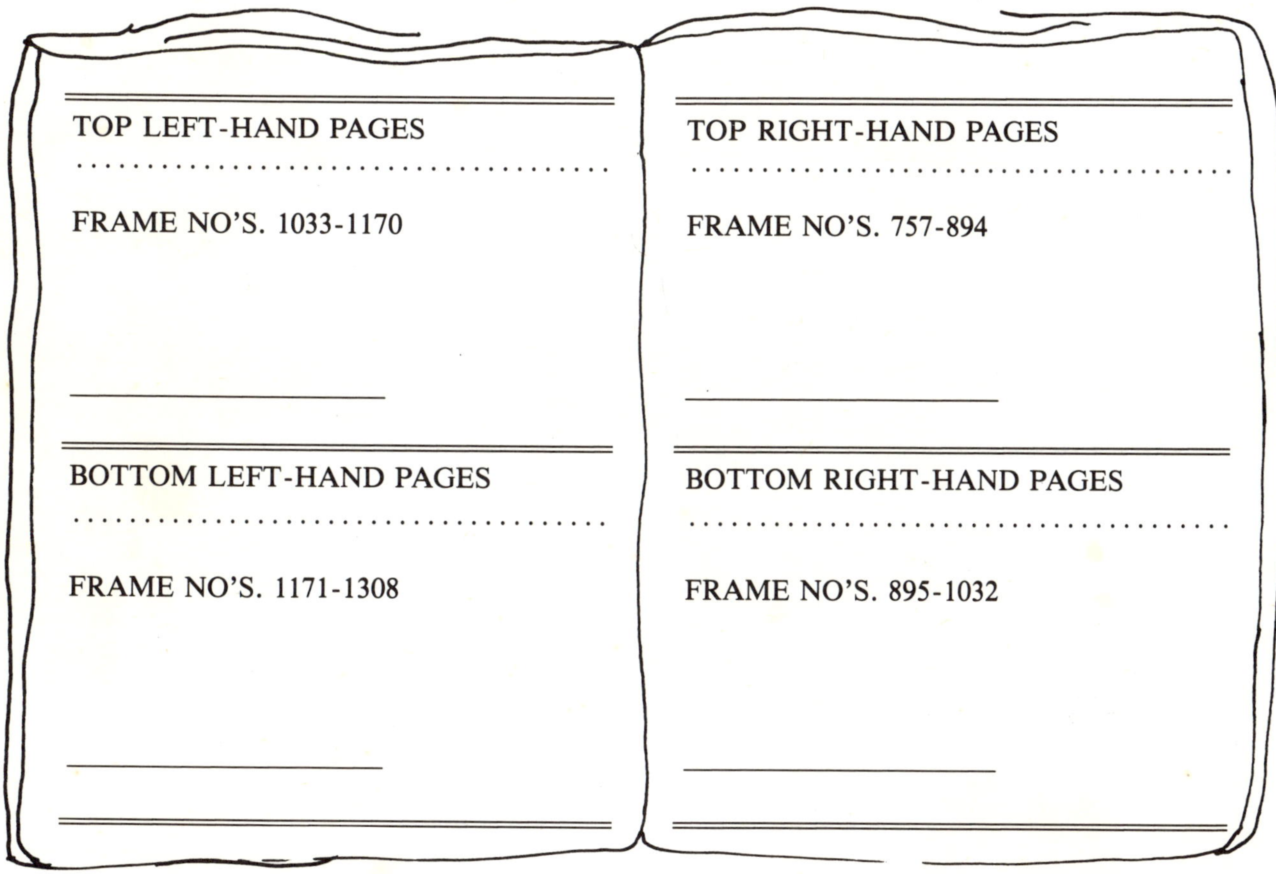

INSTRUCTIONS:

1. Decide the Frame Number you need.
2. See chart and find what *section* it is in.
3. Open book, looking at numerical sequence of that section. Find your specific frame.

EXAMPLE:

1) Find Frame 1040.
2) Section is: Top of a left-hand page.
3) Follow numerical sequence of top left-hand section and Frame 1040 is found.

A GUIDE TO THE FORMULAS

FORMULA	FRAME	PAGE
1. Base Curve Selection (B.C.S.)	859	205

Plus Lenses: B.C.S. = 6 + Spherical Equivalent

Minus Lenses: B.C.S. = $\frac{6}{2}$ + Spherical Equivalent

2. Decentration for P.D. (D.P.D.)	896	3

Monocular Horizontal = $\frac{(\text{'A' Box} + \text{dbl}) - (\text{P.D.})}{2}$

Monocular Vertical = $\frac{\text{'B' Box}}{2}$ = O.C. Height

3. Decentration for Prism (d)	907	65

$d = \frac{10 \times \Delta}{P}$

d = Decentration in millimeters
Δ = Prism
P = Power in the meridian in question.

4. Diopters (D)	1122	180

$D = \frac{1000}{f}$

D = Diopters
f = focal length in millimeters

5. Dissimilar Segments (Ds)	1045	26

$Ds = \frac{r\,(Vp + A)}{A}$

r = reading level
Vp = Vertical power
A = Add power

6. Edger Setting (E_s)	1177	14

$E_s = F_s + (P_s - 36.5)$
F_s = Finished lens size
P_s = Pattern size

7. Focal Length (f)	1111	158

$f = \frac{1000}{D}$

D = Dioptric Power

A GUIDE TO THE FORMULAS (Continued)

FORMULA	FRAME	PAGE
8. Index of Refraction	806	99
9. Jump (J)	1007	225
10. Magnification (M_t)	1090	116
11. Pantoscopic Tilt Compensation	1207	74
12. Needed Lens Blank Size (N.L.B.S.)	904	19
13. Spherical Equivalent (S.E.)	1244	148
14. Vertex Distance (V.D.) (Diopter Change)	1130	196

8. Index of Refraction

$$n = \frac{\text{speed of light in air}}{\text{speed of light in a given lens material}}$$

n = index of refraction

9. Jump (J)

$$J = \frac{dd \times dp}{10} + \frac{sd + sp}{10}$$

dd = distance decentration
dp = distance power
sd = seg decentration
sp = seg power

10. Magnification (M_t)

$M_t = M_s \times M_p$

M_t = Shape Factor × Power Factor

$$M_t = \frac{1}{1 - \frac{(t \times D)}{n}} \times \frac{1}{1 - (D_v \times h)}$$

t = thickness in meters
D = Base Curve
n = index of refraction
h = vertex distance in meters
D_v = lens power

11. Pantoscopic Tilt Compensation

Rule: Lower O.C. 1 mm. for every 2° of tilt.

12. Needed Lens Blank Size (N.L.B.S.)

N.L.B.S. = E.D. + ('A' Box + dbl) − (P.D.)

13. Spherical Equivalent (S.E.)

$$S.E. = \frac{\text{Cylinder}}{2} + \text{Sphere}$$

14. Vertex Distance (V.D.)
(Diopter Change)

$$D_c = \frac{\text{mmm.}}{1000} \times P^2$$

mmm. = millimeters moved
P = lens power

INDEX

INDEX (Continued)

INDEX (Continued)

GRACIE WANTS TO KNOW . . .

What did you think of this work? Please take a few moments to share your feelings. Your comments will be appreciated and will help with future publications.

Gracie Enterprises, Inc.
P.O. Box 506
Chula Vista, California
92012-0506

For Your Notes

For Your Notes